DrExam™ Part B MRCS OSCE Revision Guide: Book 2

Clinical Examination, Communication Skills & History Taking

Editors:

B.H. Miranda
K. Asaad
Prof. P.E.M. Butler

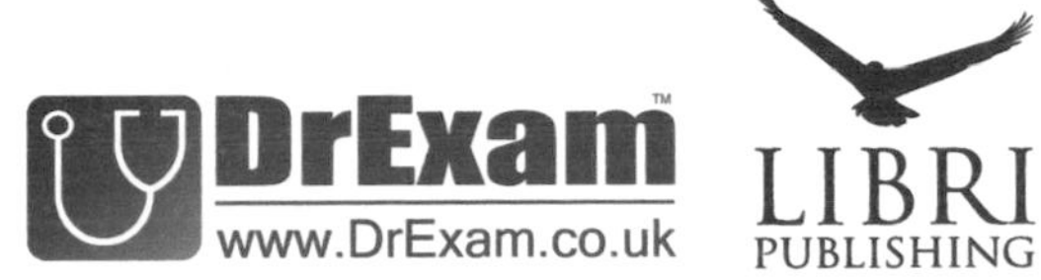

Second edition first published in 2017 by Libri Publishing

ISBN 978-1-911450-04-7

A CIP catalogue record for this book is available from The British Library

Design by Carnegie Publishing Ltd

First edition published in 2010 by Libri Publishing

Printed in the UK by Hobbs the Printers

Libri Publishing
Brunel House
Volunteer Way
Faringdon
Oxfordshire
SN7 7YR

Tel: +44 (0)845 873 3837

www.libripublishing.co.uk

CONTENTS

About the Editors......ix
Authors & Contributors......xi
Acknowledgements......xiv
Preface......xv
Dedication......xvi
Introduction (Important – Read Me!)......xvii

- How to Use this Book......xviii
- Introduction to the MRCS OSCE......xviii
- Approaching the Clinical Examination Stations, START & FINISH......xxii

SECTION A:
CLINICAL EXAMINATION STRUCTURED ROUTINES & OSCE QUESTIONS......1

SECTION A1:
LUMPS 'N' BUMPS, HEAD & NECK......1

Chapter 1: **Lumps 'n' Bumps**......3
BH Miranda, MS Soldin

The Crucial Lump Examination......4
Lumps 'n' Bumps Examination......5
OSCE Questions......8

- Differential Diagnoses......8
- Actinic Keratosis......8
- Campbell de Morgan Spot......9
- Dermatofibroma......9
- Furuncle & Carbuncle......10
- Keratoacanthoma......10
- Naevi......11
- Seborrhoeic Keratosis......12
- Neurofibroma......12
- Papilloma......13
- Pyogenic Granuloma......13

- Sebaceous Cyst 14
- Lipoma 14
- Ulcers 15

Chapter 2: Head & Neck 17
JA Joseph, BH Miranda, M Keene

Thyroid Examination 18
Thyroid Status Examination 20
Neck Lump Examination 22
Parotid Gland Examination 23
Submandibular Gland Examination 25
OSCE Questions 26

- Thyroid Embryology 26
- Goitre & Thyroid Cancer 27
- Head & Neck Lumps 30
- Head & Neck Lymph Nodes 33
- Neck Dissection 35
- Parotid Gland 36
- Tonsillitis 40
- Epistaxis 42

SECTION A2:
TRUNK & THORAX 43

Chapter 3: Breast 45
BH Miranda, D Sharpe

Breast Examination 46
OSCE Questions 49

- Fibroadenoma 49
- Excessive Breast Development 49
- Cyclical Nodularity & Mastalgia 50
- Breast Cyst 50
- Duct Ectasia 50
- Periductal Mastitis 50
- Epithelial Hyperplasia 50
- Fat Necrosis 51
- Breast Tumours 51
- Paget's Disease of the Nipple 51
- Management of Breast Disease 51

Chapter 4: Abdomen 53
BH Miranda, MJ Portou, MC Winslet

Abdominal Examination 54
OSCE Questions 59
- Clubbing 59
- Upper Gastrointestinal 60
- Hepatobiliary 62
- Spleen 66
- Kidneys 67
- Lower Gastrointestinal 69
- Rectum & Anus 73
- Common Abdominal Scars 76

Chapter 5: Herniae & Scrotum 77
BH Miranda, MJ Portou, MC Winslet

Hernia Examination 78
Scrotal Lump Examination 80
OSCE Questions 81
- Herniae 81
- Testicular Maldescent 86
- Benign Scrotal Lumps 87
- Testicular Torsion 89
- Testicular Tumours 90

Chapter 6: Stoma 93
BH Miranda , MJ Portou, MC Winslet

Stoma Examination 94
OSCE Questions 96

SECTION A3:
LIMBS, SPINE & VASCULAR 97

Chapter 7: Orthopaedics 99
S Kamalasekaran, AD Ebinesan, BH Miranda, J Saksena

Musculoskeletal Examination Tips 100
Orthopaedic Neck Examination 101
Spine Examination 104
Shoulder Examination 107
Elbow Examination 110
Hip Examination 112
Knee Examination 116

Ankle & Foot Examination 119
OSCE Questions 122
- Gait 122
- Osteoarthritis 123
- Rheumatoid Arthritis 125
- Ankylosing Spondylitis 127
- Paget's Disease of Bone 129
- Painful Shoulder 131
- Ankle & Foot Pathology 133

Chapter 8: Hands 135
K Asaad, BH Miranda, M Nicolaou, SK Al-Ghazal
Hands 136
OSCE Questions 140
- Dupuytren's Disease 140
- Ganglion 142
- Trigger Finger 143

Chapter 9: Vascular 145
M Singh, J Lorains, K Asaad, DJA Scott
Peripheral Arterial Examination 146
Varicose Veins Examination 148
OSCE Questions 150
- Arterial Insufficiency 150
- Abdominal Aortic Aneurysm 151
- Thoracic Outlet Syndrome 153
- Raynaud's Syndrome 155
- Carotid Artery Stenosis 156
- Deep Vein Thrombosis (DVT) 157
- Deep Venous Insufficiency & Venous Hypertension 158
- Varicose Veins 160
- Gangrene 161

SECTION A4:
NEUROSCIENCES 163

Chapter 10: Neuroscience 165
V Kakar, BH Miranda, J Nagaria
Abbreviated Mental Test Score 166
Mini Mental State Examination 167

Glasgow Coma Scale Assessment 168
Cranial Nerves Examination 169
Peripheral Nervous System Examination 173
DrExam's Tips for Remembering Myotomes & Nerve Roots 180
OSCE Questions 181

- Low Back Pain & Prolapsed Intervertebral Disc 181
- Cauda Equina Syndrome 183
- Head Injury 185
- Traumatic Intracranial Haemorrhage 190
- Spontaneous Intracranial Haemorrhage 192
- Stroke (CVA) 196
- Hydrocephalus 198
- CNS Infections 201
- Brain Tumours 203

Chapter 11: Upper Limb Nerves 209
BH Miranda, K Asaad, M Nicolaou, SK Al-Ghazal

Radial Nerve Examination 210
Median Nerve Examination 211
Ulnar Nerve Examination 213
OSCE Questions 216

- Radial Nerve 216
- Median Nerve 216
- Ulnar Nerve 217
- Nerve Injuries & Palsies 219

SECTION B:
COMMUNICATION SKILLS & ETHICS 221

Chapter 12: Communication Skills & Ethics 223
M Epstein, LK McMurray, BH Miranda

Introduction 224
Point Scoring 224
Key Competencies 225

- Interpersonal Skills 226
- Information Gathering 226
- Information Giving & Referral Letters 228

Ethical & Legal Principles 231

- Capacity 231
- Gillick Competence 232
- Consent 233

- Advanced Directives 235
- Organ Donation 235
- Confidentiality 236

Communication Skills OSCE Scenarios 236

- SCENARIO 1: "The angry patient" 237
- SCENARIO 2: "Breaking bad news" 240
- SCENARIO 3: "Don't tell dad about the diagnosis" 243
- SCENARIO 4: "Refusal of treatment" 245
- SCENARIO 5: "Explaining a diagnosis" 248
- SCENARIO 6: "Organ donation" 251
- SCENARIO 7: "Apologise for a mistake" 253
- SCENARIO 8: "Resuscitation decision" 256
- SCENARIO 9: "Self discharge" 258
- SCENARIO 10: "Consent to a trial" 261

SECTION C:
HISTORY TAKING 263

Chapter 13: Structured History 265
A Ebinesan, BH Miranda

Structured History 266
Presenting Complaint 266
History of Presenting Complaint 266
Past Medical & Surgical History 268
Drug History 268
Family History 268
Social History 268
Activities of Daily Living 269
Systems Review 270

Abbreviations 271

Index 275

ABOUT THE EDITORS

Ben Miranda ALCM, BSc, MBBS (Lond), MRCS (Eng), PhD

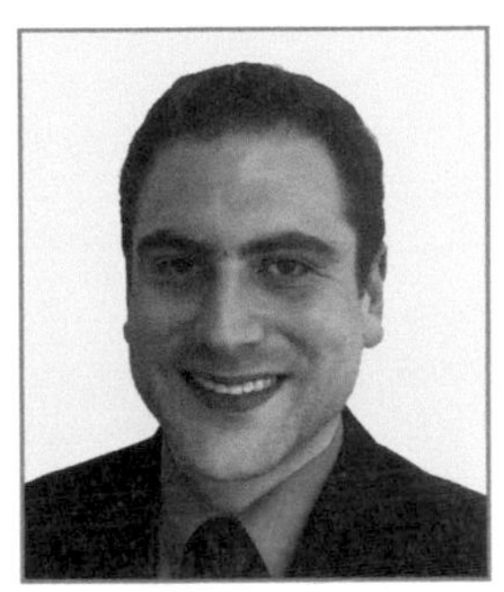

Ben is a Specialty Trainee (ST) Registrar on the London Deanery Plastic Surgery & Burns Training Rotation. He was previously a Research Registrar at the Plastic Surgery & Burns Research Unit, University of Bradford. His research interest in hair follicle biology & growth control led him to complete a PhD within three years. Having graduated from the Royal Free & University College Hospital School of Medicine (London) in 2004, he has now won 14 academic prizes & awards, primarily at postgraduate level. He has 35 published / accepted journal papers, features & books, including a front cover publication in the *British Journal of Dermatology* on part of his PhD research & 50 international / national presentations at high-end conferences. Ben has had training exposure to a wide variety of surgical specialities, including A&E, Burns, ENT, Gastrointestinal, Neurosurgery, Plastic Surgery, Urology & Vascular Surgery.

Ben's passion for education developed since 1998, when he began teaching Mathematics to GCSE & A-Level students. He continued this throughout medical school & in 2006 was drafted to teach Royal Free & University College Hospital School of Medicine MBBS finalists. In 2007 he helped to establish DrExam as a leading provider of postgraduate surgical education, in association with & in support of the Plastic Surgery & Burns Research Unit. His dedication to surgical education & the future progress of surgery has been proven by his many extracurricular activities. These include integral participation in the well-publicised £100,000 fundraising appeal for the Research Unit's 25th anniversary in 2010.

Kamil Asaad BSc (Lond), MB ChB, MRCS (Eng), MPhil

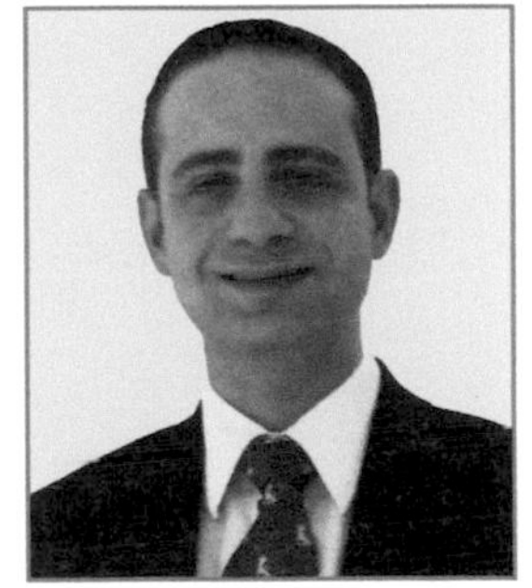

Kamil is a Plastic Surgery Specialty Trainee (ST) who graduated from Leeds University Medical School in 1999 & undertook an intercalated BSc at Imperial College School of Medicine (London) in 1997. During this time he researched antigen-presenting cells in inflammatory bowel disease at the internationally renowned St Mark's Hospital. He has previously been a Research Registrar, completing his MPhil placement in 2007 at the Plastic Surgery & Burns Research Unit, University of Bradford. His research interest here was the structural variability of skin at different sites of the body, relating this to scarring potential & he developed a new histological stain. He has 11 academic prizes & awards,15 publications & 30 international / national presentations.

Kamil has maintained an active interest in teaching since qualifying. He has regularly taught on DrExam MRCS revision courses since 2007, having helped design & establish the OSCE course in response to the changes in the MRCS examination. Kamil has had training exposure to a wide variety of surgical specialities & several years experience in Plastic Surgery & Burns. He has been key in fundraising for the Plastic Surgery & Burns Research Unit in Bradford during its 20th & 21st anniversaries. He has worked as an expert reviewer for the London Student Journal of Medicine as well as a Medical Consultant for several film & television projects.

Professor Peter EM Butler MD, FRCSI, FRCS, FRCS (Plast)

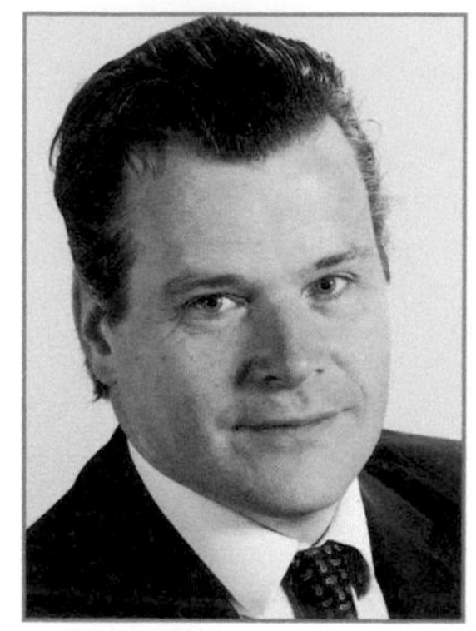

Professor Butler is a fellow of the Royal College of Surgeons in Ireland & England. He trained in Plastic Surgery in Dublin followed by a research fellowship at Harvard Medical School (USA), completing the Plastic Surgery Fellowship of the Royal College of Surgeons in 1998.

Professor Butler is a council member of the British Association of Plastic Surgeons & chairman of the Research & Education Committee. He has over 100 Plastic Surgery publications & has published many book chapters, with international presentations in the USA, Canada, Italy, France & Mexico. He has an active clinical & laboratory based research program & is world renowned for his work, leading the UK Facial Transplant team. He has received awards from the New England Society of Plastic & Reconstructive Surgeons, the American Society of Plastic & Reconstructive Surgeons, the Plastic Surgery Research Council (USA) & the British Association of Plastic Surgeons.

He is a Consultant Plastic Surgeon & Honorary Senior Lecturer at the Royal Free & University College Hospitals (London) & a Consultant in Plastic Surgery at the Massachusetts General Hospital, Boston, USA. In 2005, he was appointed Visiting Professor to the Divisions of Plastic Surgery, University of Pittsburgh & MD Anderson Cancer Centre, Texas.

AUTHORS & CONTRIBUTORS

Mr Sharif Kaf Al-Ghazal MS, MD, FRCS
Consultant Plastic Surgeon
Bradford Teaching Hospitals
Honorary Senior Lecturer
School of Medicine, University of Leeds

Dr John Annaradnam MB BS, MRCGP
General Practitioner
The Southgate Surgery, London

Mr Kamil Asaad BSc, MB ChB, MRCS, MPhil
Plastic Surgery Registrar
St Thomas' Hospital London

Mr Omar Baldo MBBS, MRCS
Specialty Registrar Urology
Yorkshire Deanery

Dr Heike I Bauer
Consultant Dermatologist
Bradford Teaching Hospitals NHS Foundation Trust

Carly Betton MA, BA (Hons), MIMI, RMIP
Senior Clinical Photographer
University Hospitals Birmingham NHS Foundation Trust

Mr Waseem Bhat MuDr, MA, MRCS
Clinical Fellow Plastic Surgery
Castle Hill Hospital, Cottingham

Wendy Birch BSc (Hons), MSc, MBIE, LIAS
Anatomist & Dissection Room Manager
Research Department of Cell and Developmental Biology
University College London Medical School

Mr Quamar MK Bismil MB ChB (Hons), MRCS, Dip SEM, MFSEM, FRCS (Tr & Orth)
Specialty Registrar Trauma & Orthopaedics
London Deanery

Professor Peter EM Butler MD, FRCSI, FRCS, FRCS (Plast)
Professor of Plastic Surgery & Honorary Senior Lecturer
Royal Free & University College Hospitals London

Laurence Clarke MBIE, LIAS, FAAPT
Senior Anatomy Technician
Research Department of Cell and Developmental Biology
University College London Medical School

Paul Creasey BSc MIMI, RMIP
Senior Clinical Photographer
Bradford Teaching Hospitals NHS Trust

Antony Dook BSc, MIMI, RMIP
Chief Clinical Photographer
Bradford Teaching Hospitals NHS Trust

Mr AD Ebinesan MB ChB, MRCS (Eng)
Specialist Registrar in Trauma & Orthopaedics
North Western Rotation

Dr Marc Epstein BSc, MBBS, MRCGP, MRCP
General Practitioner

Ms Edwina Ewart BSc (Hons), MBChB, MRCS (Ed)
MD Research Registar
Northern Lincolnshire & Goole Hospitals NHS Trust

Carol Fleming BSc, FIMI, RMIP
Principal Clinical Photographer & Medical Illustration Manager
Bradford Teaching Hospitals NHS Foundation Trust

Mr Ivan Foo FRCS Eng (Plast), FRCS Ed
Consultant Plastic & Reconstructive Surgeon
Bradford Teaching Hospitals NHS Foundation Trust

Miss Sheila Fraser MB ChB MRCS
Specialty Registrar General Surgery
Yorkshire Deanery

Dr Brian Geffin MB BCh, MRCGP
General Practitioner
The Southgate Surgery, London

Dr Brijanand Sharma Ghoorun MD, FRCA
Consultant ITU & Trauma Anaesthetist
Huddersfield Royal Infirmary

Katherine Grice BA, MIMI, RMIP
Senior Clinical Photographer
Bradford Teaching Hospitals NHS Trust

Dr Ayshea Hameeduddin MBBS, BA (Hons) Med Journalism, FRCR
Specialist Trainee in Radiology
Royal Free Hospital, London

Dr Brian Holloway MRCS, FRCR
Consultant Radiologist
Royal Free Hospital, London

Mr Jonathan A Joseph BSc, MBBS, MRCS, DOHNS
Specialist Registrar in ENT
Oxford Deanery

Mr Vishal Kakar BSc, MBBS (Lond), MRCS (Eng)
Specialty Registrar Neurosurgery
Northern Ireland Deanery

Mr Senthil Kamalasekaran MB ChB, MS (Orth), MRCS
Trauma & Orthopaedics Registrar
Barnet & Chase Farm Hospitals NHS Trust

Professor Simon P Kay FRCS, FRCS (Plast), FRCS Ed (Hon)
Professor of Plastic & Reconstructive Surgery & Surgery of the Hand
Leeds Teaching Hospitals NHS Trust

Mr Malcolm Keene MBBS, FRCS
Consultant ENT Surgeon
Barts and the London NHS Trust

Mr R Linforth MD, FRCS Ed, FRCS (Gen Surg)
Consultant Breast & Oncoplastic Surgeon
Bradford Teaching Hospitals NHS Foundation Trust

Dr KM London
Consultant Dermatologist
Bradford Teaching Hospitals NHS Foundation Trust

Ms Joanna Lorains BSc, MB ChB, MRCS
Specialty Registrar General Surgery
North Western Deanery

Dr Anmol Malhotra BSc (Hons), MRCP, FRCR
Consultant Radiologist
Royal Free Hospital, London

Mr JC May MB, BCh, FRCS Ed (Gen)
Consultant General Surgeon
Bradford Teaching Hospitals NHS Foundation Trust

Ms Laura K McMurray BSc, PGCMCH, PGCCBT, PGDipCBT
Psychological Therapist
Isllington Psychological Assessment & Treatment Service, London

Mr Benjamin H Miranda ALCM, BSc, MBBS (Lond), MRCS (Eng)
Plastic Surgery & Burns Research Registrar
Plastic Surgery & Burns Research Unit
University of Bradford

Mr Jabir Nagaria MBBS, FRCS (Surgical Neurology)
Consultant Neurosurgeon
Royal Victoria Hospital
Belfast

Mr Marios Nicolaou BMedSci, BMBS, MRCS, PhD
Specialty Registrar in Plastic Surgery & Burns
Oxford Deanery

Dr Selva Nithiyananthan MB BS, MRCP, DipMedRehab, MRCGP
General Practitioner
The Southgate Surgery, London

Dr Stephen Oakey MBBS, FRCA
Consultant in Anaesthesia & Burns Critical Care
St Andrew's Centre for Plastic Surgery & Burns
Broomfield Hospital, Chelmsford

Mr Kanak K Patel FDS, RCPS, FRCS (OMFS)
Consultant Oral & Maxillofacial Surgeon
Bradford Teaching Hospitals NHS Foundation Trust

Mr Mark James Portou MB ChB (Hons), MRCS
Specialty Registrar in General Surgery
London Deanery

Mr N Rhodes FFDRCS, FRCS (Plast)
Consultant Plastic & Reconstructive Surgeon
Bradford Teaching Hospitals NHS Foundation Trust

Mr J Saksena BMSc (Hons), MB ChB, MRCS, FRCS (Tr&Orth)
Consultant Orthopaedic & Trauma Surgeon
The Whittington Hospital London

Professor DJA Scott MD, MB ChB, FRCS, FEBVS
Professor of Vascular Surgery
Division of Cardiovascular and Diabetes Research
Leeds Institute of Genetics, Health and Therapeutics

Professor David T Sharpe OBE, MA, Bchir, FRCS
Professor of Plastic & Reconstructive Surgery
Plastic Surgery & Burns Research Unit Director
University of Bradford

Mr Masha Singh MBBS, BSc, MRCS
Department of General Surgery
Bradford Royal Infirmary

Mr Niroshan Sivathasan BSc, MBBS, MRCS (Eng)
Registrar in Plastic Surgery
Broomfield Hospital, Chelmsford

Sarah Slade BA (Hons), MIMI, RMIP
Clinical Photographer
Bradford Teaching Hospitals NHS Trust

Mr Mark S Soldin MB ChB, FCS (SA), FRCS (Plast)
Consultant Plastic & Reconstructive Surgeon
St George's Healthcare NHS Trust London

Mr M A Steward FRCS (Ed)
Consultant Colorectal & General Surgeon
Bradford Teaching Hospitals NHS Foundation Trust

Mr D N Sutton BDS, FRCDS (Ed), FRCS (Ed), FRCS (Eng)
Consultant Oral & Maxillofacial Surgeon
Bradford Teaching Hospitals NHS Foundation Trust

Mr Michael J Timmons MA, MChir, FRCS
Consultant Plastic & Reconstructive Surgeon
Bradford Teaching Hospitals NHS Foundation Trust

Professor Desmond J Tobin PhD, FRCPath, FIBiol
Director of the Centre for Skin Sciences
Professor of Cell Biology
Assoc. Dean of Research & Knowledge Transfer
University of Bradford

Mr David A L Watt MB ChB, FRCS (Plast)
Consultant Plastic & Reconstructive Surgeon
Bradford Teaching Hospitals NHS Foundation Trust

Professor Marc C Winslet MS, FRCS (Ed), FRCS (Eng), MEWI
Professor of Surgery, Head of Department
Chairman of Division of Surgery & Interventional Science
School of Medicine
Faculty of Biomedical Science
University College London

Dr A L Wright BMedSci (Hons), LRCP, MRCS, MB ChB, FRCP
Consultant Dermatologist & Lead Clinician
Bradford Teaching Hospitals NHS Foundation Trust

'The Anatomy Dissection Team'
Rachel Eyre, Rebecca Gayner, Emma Williams, James Davis, Lucy Collison, David Reynolds, Alexander, Morton, Gopigia Thana-Balasundaram, Timothy Chan, Oliver White, Zoya Georgieva, James Lewis, Brett Packham, Kevin Cao, Radoslaw Rippel, Donald Leith

ACKNOWLEDGEMENTS

'Putting this MRCS OSCE revision guide book series together has been one of our most challenging & rewarding experiences to date.

We could not have done it without the help of our teachers past & present, our co-contributors – Professors, Consultants, other professional colleagues or even our students...

... BUT...

In particular we would like to thank the following people in no particular order: Mrs Gladys Miranda, Mr David Miranda, Dr Issa Asaad & Dr Lillian Asaad.

Mums & Dads we thank you & will never forget your unconditional love & support.'

Ben & Kamil

PREFACE

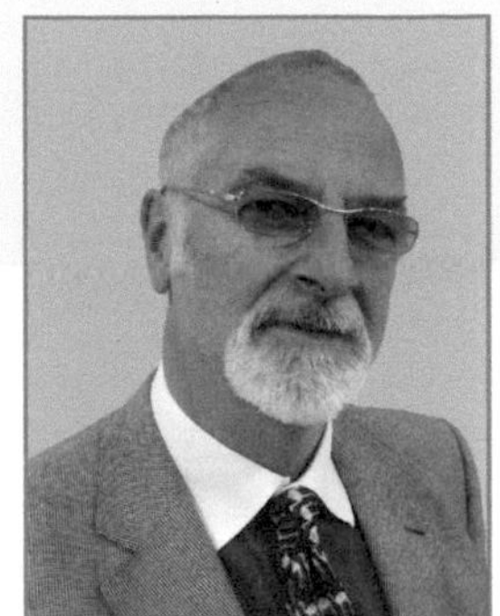

The DrExam MRCS Part B OSCE revision guide series adopts an innovative approach which addresses the needs of candidates for the revised MRCS OSCE exam. The authors have tackled subjects that are common, complicated or important, according to the new syllabus. This was only achievable through the collaborative efforts of 6 professors, 26 consultants & 24 specialists from across the United Kingdom.

DrExam has several years of experience in teaching MRCS candidates on revision courses that have evolved & adapted to the changes in the exam. These highly successful courses (www.DrExam.co.uk) have become internationally attended & this book series has developed following high candidate success rates & positive feedback about the teaching quality, knowledge imparted & detailed course handouts provided.

What differentiates these books from others is that they are targeted specifically to the OSCE, in structured question-answer format throughout, illustrated by fantastic high-resolution colour images that were contributed by anatomists, radiologists, clinical photographers & medical illustrators. Each chapter, or sections within a chapter, has been written or verified by specialists within the field.

Topics covered in detail in Book 1 include: Radiology, Critical Care, Physiology, Anatomy, Surgical Pathology, Operative Surgery & Surgical Skills, Bones & Soft Tissues, Endocrinology, Oncology & Surgical Technology.

Topics covered in detail in Book 2 include: Clinical Examination Protocols, Lumps 'n' Bumps, Head & Neck, Trunk & Thorax, Limbs Spine & Vascular, Neurosciences, Communication Skills, Ethics & History Taking. In addition, clinical examination is taught not only with written words & pictures, but also with a DVD containing all major examination routines. This allows the candidate to pick up 'nuances' of clinical examination that are not readily communicated through still images alone.

The Bradford Burns & Plastic Surgery Research Unit evolved following the Bradford City Football Club stadium fire disaster in 1985. Twenty five percent of the royalties from this series will be donated to the unit so that it may continue to make a valuable contribution to skin sciences research & future patient care. Ben Miranda & Kamil Asaad were Research Registrars at the unit & it is rewarding to see their continuing contribution.

The DrExam series is the most colourful, complete & structured MRCS OSCE revision guide to be released on the market to date & I thank all those who were involved in making this project a success. It will not only be of great value to any MRCS OSCE candidate, but also to training surgeons, doctors, medical practitioners & students who are required to revise these vital core subjects.

Professor David T Sharpe OBE

This book is dedicated to the memory of the 56 who died, 270 who were injured & thousands more who were affected by the Bradford City Football Club stadium fire disaster on 11th May 1985.

INTRODUCTION
(IMPORTANT - READ ME!)

BH Miranda
K Asaad
PEM Butler

CONTENTS

How to Use this Book

Introduction to the MRCS OSCE

- OSCE Exam Overview
- OSCE Structure
- OSCE Disciplines
- OSCE Speciality Themes
- Point Scoring
- OSCE Domains
- What to Wear!

Approaching the Clinical Examination Stations, Start & Finish

- Start
- Clinical Examination
- Finish

Please read the following sections carefully, they provide the candidate with vital tips regarding the use of this book, accompanying DVD, how to approach the MRCS OSCE & maintain good clinical practice in the future.

HOW TO USE THIS BOOK

- The primary objective of this book is to present **structured clinical examination routines that are reproducible in the MRCS OSCE & in everyday clinical practice**. These routines represent a thorough framework, reviewed by Professors, Consultants & Specialists in their respective fields, which may be modified to accommodate normal variations in clinical practice. *These appear at the beginning of each chapter.*
- The **accompanying clinical examination tutorial DVD** also covers these examination routines & should be used in conjunction with the routines in this book.
- An additional objective is to provide the candidate with **questions & structured / categorised answers relating to clinical topics that are commonly asked during the MRCS OSCE & in everyday clinical practice**. *These appear at the end of each chapter.*
- Candidates are advised to **learn & consistently practice these routines**, so that they may be reproduced almost involuntarily, in order to become competent clinicians! This may be achieved via use of books, attendance at courses & on the wards / in clinic.
- **To cover the remaining half of the MRCS OSCE syllabus**, there is a sister volume: **DrExam Part B MRCS OSCE Revision Guide: Book 1** *Applied Surgical Science & Critical Care, Anatomy & Surgical Pathology, Surgical Skills & Patient Safety.*
- **There are two Courses** also available to complement these books. Candidates can find these by visiting **www.DrExam.co.uk.**

INTRODUCTION TO THE MRCS OSCE

Note: The OSCE has recently changed format again & is likely to do so in the future. These changes are mostly to do with the format / marking scheme of the examination, however the knowledge & skill level required to succeed remains largely unaffected. The following information should be used as a general guide to the OSCE format, which should be confirmed by the candidate via contacting The Royal College of Surgeons.

OSCE Exam Overview

- Anatomy & surgical pathology
- Applied surgical science & critical care
- Clinical & procedural skills
- Communication skills

OSCE Structure

- 18 stations (possibility of several additional preparation stations)

OSCE Disciplines

Applied Surgical Science & Critical Care, Anatomy & Surgical Pathology, Surgical Skills & Patient Safety (DrExam Part B MRCS OSCE Revision Guide: Book 1)

- Applied surgical science & critical care
- Anatomy & surgical pathology
- Operative surgery & surgical skills
- Principles of surgery & patient safety

Clinical Examination, Communication Skills & History taking (DrExam Part B MRCS OSCE Revision Guide: Book 2)

- Clinical examination
- Communication skills
- History taking

OSCE Speciality Themes

The candidate will be required to have knowledge across the following:

- Head & neck
- Trunk & thorax
- Limbs & spine (including vascular)
- Neuroscience

Point Scoring

- Each station carries 20 marks
- The maximum achievable score for the 18 OSCE stations is 360
- An overall rating is additionally allocated by the examiner at each station as follows:
  1. Fail
  2. Borderline fail
  3. Borderline pass
  4. Pass
- A minimum pass mark will then be calculated based on the station marks & overall rating at each station.
- In addition to the minimum pass mark, the candidate must achieve a minimum level of competence in OSCE disciplines (see above) & OSCE domains (see below).

OSCE Domains

- 4 domains of knowledge, skill, competence & professional attributes are tested throughout the OSCE.
- These domains are intrinsic to good surgical practice.
- Domains may be tested throughout the 18 stations of the OSCE.
- It is therefore important to consider these 4 domains at every station throughout the OSCE.

Domain	Notes
Clinical Knowledge	Understand, process & apply knowledge in a clinical setting.
Clinical & Technical Skill	Apply knowledge, awareness & skill to generate differential diagnoses & aid investigation of a clinical problem. Perform surgical tasks that require manual dexterity, hand-eye coordination & visual-spatial awareness.
Communication	Process information, identify what is important & convey it to others clearly, by engaging a patient, carer or colleague during a consultation.
Professionalism	Demonstrate effective judgement & decision making by processing & addressing all appropriate information prior to formulating a plan. Identify rapidly deteriorating conditions & think laterally to maximise efficiency. Show awareness of limitations & seek help when appropriate. Accommodate changing information to manage a clinical problem. Anticipate & plan in advance. Prioritise effectively & demonstrate good time management.

What to Wear!

Modern infection control practices have precipitated a review of dress code for the OSCE as follows:

- Arms bare below the elbow
- No jewellery on hands or wrists except wedding rings / bands
- No ties or dangling clothing.

Female candidates may wish to present themselves as follows:

- Smart haircut with tied-back hair (if long)
- Smart blouse, sleeves rolled up to above the elbows
- Smart skirt / trousers
- Smart & comfortable shoes (not open)
- Minimal jewellery & makeup.

Male candidates may wish to present themselves as follows:

- Smart haircut
- Smart shirt, sleeves rolled up to above the elbows.
- No tie
- Smart trousers
- Smart & comfortable shoes
- No jewellery other than a wedding ring / band.

APPROACHING THE CLINICAL EXAMINATION STATIONS, START & FINISH!

It is important to conduct yourself throughout the OSCE stations, in a manner that is appropriate to real clinical settings. It is therefore important to establish a good rapport with your 'patient' & examiner by using effective communication strategies *(see communication skills chapter).* Remember to be calm, clear & calculative when talking to both the examiner & patient. Never 'bleat' out an answer that hasn't been thought through systematically. It doesn't hurt to smile & be friendly either!

Passing the clinical examination stations requires a systematic approach that appears almost involuntary. Examiners are unlikely to interrupt or prompt the candidate, so it is vital to display an award-winning performance. The best way for the candidate to ensure that they perform successfully during clinical examination stations, is to practise, practise & practise beforehand! This will ensure that the candidate develops a structured & systematic approach that is easily identifiable to the examiner.

A structured & systematic clinical examination performance may be thought of in 3 stages:

1. START

2. CLINICAL EXAMINATION

3. FINISH

It is also useful to have a standard introduction strategy for the start & finish of the clinical examination stations.

Memory:	START:	FINISH:
	I Want PC PEG	*To Happily Wave at Safe Drivers*
	Introduction	**Thank Patient**
	Wash Hands	**Help Patient Dress**
	Permission	**Wash Hands**
	Chaperone	**Summary**
	Position	**Differential Diagnosis**
	Exposure	
	General Inspection	

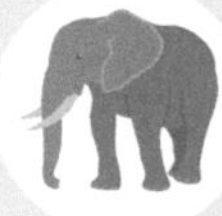

START

Introduction, Wash Hands & Permission:

It is important to have a standard introduction strategy that is easily recallable under the influence of OSCE nerves! This should also include obtaining consent for the examination & hand washing. It is important to remember to wash your hands before & after each case. Here is an example opening statement:

> *'Hello, my name is Dr X. I am one of the candidates for today's examination. Is it alright for me to examine your head / neck / chest / back / hip / legs etc?'*

You may be required to communicate your findings to the examiner as you go along. If so you can add:

> *'... & talk to the examiner as I go along?'*

You may have to adjust your introduction according to the scenario as follows:

> **Scenario: You are the CT2 doctor on call & have been asked to see Mrs Deyton who has a blocked catheter. You are informed that she is in pain & you arrive at her bedside. Begin the consultation.**
>
> *'Hello Mrs Deyton, my name is Dr X. I am the CT2 doctor on call & I understand that you have a blocked catheter. Are you in any pain at all? ...'*

Chaperone:

All sensitive examination areas require a chaperone e.g. breast & scrotum. It is also important to maintain patient dignity via the use of a bed sheet. You should communicate to the examiner that you are considering these points, by interacting with the patient:

> *'I will need a chaperone in order to examine your breasts. Is this alright?'*
>
> *'Yes doctor!'*
>
> *'Thank you, we will get some sheets to keep you covered up.'*

Position & Exposure:

Remember that each clinical examination routine requires careful consideration of the relevant position & exposure of the patient. These will be discussed at the relevant **START** sections of the structured routines throughout this book.

General Inspection:

General inspection precedes every clinical examination routine. Stand a step away from the foot of the bed, in line with the patient's midline. If the patient is sitting in a chair & it is appropriate, stand opposite the patient. In this position, with your **hands behind your back**, comment on:

1. **The general health of the patient:**

   'Standing at the end of the bed, the patient looks comfortable at rest...'

2. **Peripheral markers of disease:**

   '... & there are no peripheral markers of disease.'

Comment on peripheral markers of disease by looking purposefully around the patient & bedside. Peripheral markers of disease may be classified as follows:

Classification	Examples
General Surgical	Cannula, Catheter, Drain & Fluid Line
Breast	Prosthesis & Support Bra
Cardiovascular	Cardiac Monitor, Cigarettes & ECG Leads
Gastrointestinal	Commode, Kidney Dish & Stoma Bag
Neurological	Hearing Aid & Walking Stick
Orthopaedic	Crutches, Plaster Cast, Prosthesis & Walking Stick
Respiratory	Cigarettes, Inhaler, Peak Flow Meter & Pulse Oximeter Probe
Vascular	Cigarettes, Compression Bandage & Prosthesis

CLINICAL EXAMINATION

Move to the relevant examination position that is specific to each examination routine. These will be discussed in the relevant **START** sections of the structured routines throughout this book. **Remember to conduct all examinations, which require the patient to be on an examination couch, standing to the right side of the patient.**

FINISH

Thank Patient & Wash Hands:

Thank the patient for their time & wash your hands. **It is important to remember to wash your hands before & after each case.**

Summary & Differential Diagnosis:

Summarise the relevant positive & negative findings from your clinical examination of the patient. Your findings should be reported in a similar order & format to your clinical examination routine i.e. inspection, palpation, percussion & auscultation. Offer a differential diagnosis that is classified, in a similar manner to those that are presented throughout Books 1 & 2.

SECTION A: CLINICAL EXAMINATION STRUCTURED ROUTINES & OSCE QUESTIONS

SECTION A1: LUMPS 'N' BUMPS, HEAD & NECK

CHAPTER 1
LUMPS 'N' BUMPS

BH Miranda
MS Soldin

CHAPTER CONTENTS

The Crucial Lump Examination

Lumps 'n' Bumps Examination

Ulcer Examination

OSCE Questions *(also see book 1 oncology chapter for BCC, SCC & melanoma)*

- Differential Diagnoses
- Actinic Keratosis
- Campbell de Morgan Spot
- Dermatofibroma
- Furuncle & Carbuncle
- Keratoacanthoma
- Naevi
- Seborrhoeic Keratosis
- Neurofibroma
- Papilloma
- Pyogenic Granuloma
- Sebaceous Cyst
- Lipoma
- Ulcers

THE CRUCIAL LUMP EXAMINATION

The examination of a lump may be important in all surgical specialities:

Speciality	Examples
ENT	Head & Neck Cancer
General Surgery	Organomegaly
Orthopaedics	Bone Tumours
Plastic Surgery	Benign Lumps & Skin Cancer
Urology	Bladder & Penile Cancer
Vascular Surgery	Aneurysms & Varicose Veins

For this reason in the OSCE, it is vital for the candidate to demonstrate an examination protocol that covers all the important clinical features of the lump. The protocol presented in this chapter is universal, so it is important to remember that some parts may not be relevant to all lumps e.g. do not auscultate a lump in the neck for bowel sounds!

LUMPS 'N' BUMPS EXAMINATION

START: Ensure adequate exposure of the lump & surrounding region:

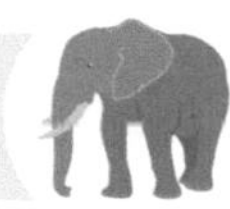

Memory: The 6 x S's of inspection.

INSPECTION	Interpretation
Site	Anatomical location e.g. dorsum of the right hand or anterior triangle of the neck.
Size	Approximate size of base e.g. 3cm x 2cm.
Shape	Approximate shape of base & indicate dimensions e.g. hemispherical & protuberant.
Symmetry	Remember that lumps may be asymmetrical e.g. melanoma, symmetrical about the midline e.g. goitre or symmetrical about their own axis e.g. cyst.
Skin	Comment on the overlying & surrounding skin e.g. erythematous, punctum visible or ulcerated.
Scars	Comment on the presence of scars that may be indicative of previous surgery.

Ask about pain.

Feel for temperature changes with the back of your hand.

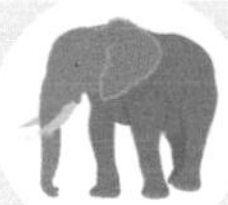

Memory: 'SEC FFP TR' or Sister Entered Clinic, Frowning at Frightened Peter's Terrible Result

PALPATION	Interpretation
Surface	Rough or smooth.
Edge	Irregular, infiltrative or well defined.
Consistency	Comment if the consistency is: • **Hard** (feels like the nasal bridge). • **Firm** (feels like the nasal tip). • **Soft** (feels like the nares).
Fixed	Comment if the lump is: • **Fixed to skin** (the skin will not move freely over the lump). • **Fixed to underlying tissue** (the lump will not move freely over underlying tissue). • **Fixed to the muscle surface** (the lump becomes more prominent with contraction of underlying muscle). • **Within muscle** (the lump will become less prominent with muscle contraction).
Fluctuant	**Paget's Sign:** Use the index & middle finger of 1 hand to stabilise the base of the lump. Press the middle of the lump with the index finger of the other hand. A lump is fluctuant if the edges press / spill over the tops of the stabilising fingers e.g. cyst. This should be done in 2 planes.
Pulsatile / Expansile	Use the index fingers of both hands, in parallel, to demonstrate. Place a finger on each edge of the lump. Pulsatile lumps will move your fingers up & down in a vertical plan e.g. lump overlying an artery or a well-vascularised tumour. Expansile lumps will move your fingers outward & inward in a radial plane e.g. aneurysm.
Transilluminable	Shine a torch into one side of the lump & look at the contralateral side. Fluid-filled lumps will glow brightly on the contralateral side e.g. cyst.
Reducible	Always ask a patient to reduce their lump first, then ask if you may reduce it e.g. hernia.

It may not be appropriate to percuss some lumps e.g. scrotal hernias.

PERCUSSION	Interpretation
Sternum	Fluid-filled lumps may have a fluid thrill or be stony dull to percussion.

It may not be appropriate to auscultate for bowel sounds or bruits in all lumps e.g. neck lumps where you would listen for bruits, not bowel sounds. Remember to auscultate for bowel sounds in all scrotal lumps that may be hernias containing bowel loops.

AUSCULTATION	Interpretation
Lump	Auscultate for bowel sounds or bruits.

COMPLETION	Interpretation
Lymphadenopathy	Check draining regional lymph nodes. Compare with contralateral side where possible. Watch for normal structures that may be mistaken for lymphadenopathy e.g. the greater horn of the hyoid bone, a prominent transverse arch of the atlas & the submandibular gland.
Neurovascular Status	Ensure no encroachment on nerves or vessels by performing a distal neurological & vascular examination.
General Examination	Lumps may be a cause or consequence of metastasis so it is important to perform an appropriate general examination e.g. breast lumps should prompt an abdominal, respiratory & spinal examination.
Cosmetic & Quality of Life	Establish if the patient is affected by the appearance of the lump & whether it affects their quality of life in any way.

FINISH:

Ulcers

Ulcers are clinically examined like all lumps, however it is important that the following features are also addressed when inspecting ulcers:

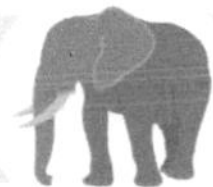

Memory: Ulcers have BEDS

Ulcer Inspection	Interpretation	
Base	Granulation Tissue, Slough	
Edge	**Sloping:**	Traumatic & Venous Ulcers
	Punched:	Arterial Ulcers
	Undermined:	TB
	Rolled:	BCC
	Everted:	SCC & Marjolin's Ulcer
Discharge	Serous, Sanguinous, Serosanguinous, Purulent	
Structures Visible	Muscles, Vessels, Bone	

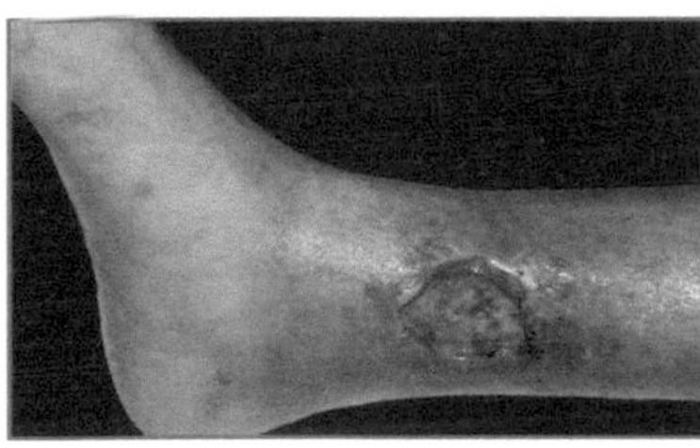

Fig 1.1: Venous ulceration of the gaiter area & medial malleolus of the right lower limb. There is healthy granulation tissue at the ulcer base, with some slough. There is associated haemosiderin deposition & lipodermatosclerosis.

OSCE QUESTIONS

Q: What are the differential diagnoses for a lump?

The differentials for any lump are classified by location as follows:

Location	Examples		
Cutaneous	**Benign:**	Actinic Keratosis, Campbell de Morgan Spots, Dermatofibroma, Keratoacanthoma, Naevus, Seborrhoeic Keratosis	
	Malignant:	**Epidermal:**	BCC, SCC, Melanoma
		Dermal:	DFSP, Malignant Fibrous Histiocytoma
Subcutaneous	Cyst		
Fat	Lipoma		
Artery	Aneurysm		
Vein	Varicosity		
Nerve	Neuroma		
Lymph Node	Lymphadenopathy		
Muscle	Tumour		
Bone	Tumour, Malunited Fracture, Osteoma		
Anatomical Region	Ganglion (dorsum of hand), Liver (right hypochondrium), Hernias (groin) etc.		

Q: What is actinic keratosis?

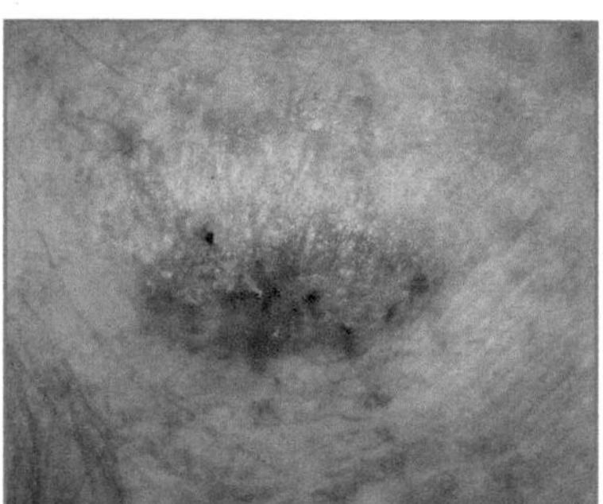

Fig 1.2: **Actinic keratosis.**

This is the most common pre-malignant lesion of the skin, caused by chronic sun damage. Actinic keratoses are common on the face & present as rough white patches stuck onto an erythematous base. Histology reveals thickening of the keratin (hyperkeratosis) & prickle cell (acanthosis) layers of the skin, increased cell mitoses & dysplasia. An actinic keratosis may be considered as a SCC *in situ* as 10–15% may progress to SCC.

Q: What treatment options are available for actinic keratosis?

Like all treatment options, they may be classified as conservative, medical & surgical:

Conservative	Medical	Surgical
Sun Protection	Diclofenac Sodium Gel (Solaraze™)	Cautery
(prevention is the best treatment)	5- Fluorouracil Cream	Cryosurgery
	Cryotherapy	Laser
		Surgical Excision

Q: What are Campbell de Morgan spots?

These are cherry haemangiomas formed by a proliferation of dilated venules. They are more common with increasing age & are seen as small, bright red papules on the skin. Treatment is conservative, however cryotherapy, curettage & shave excision are also options.

Q: What is a dermatofibroma?

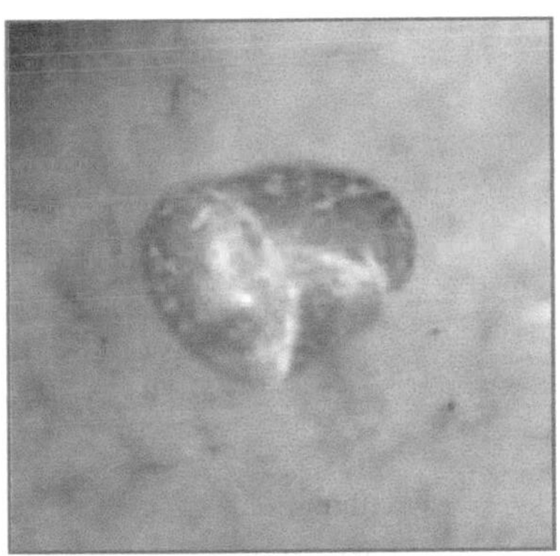

Fig 1.3: Dermatofibroma.

A benign neoplasm of dermal fibroblasts or 'histiocytoma'. A history of trauma is usually present e.g. insect bite. The lesion is a firm papule, usually 5–8 mm in size & roughly circular within the dermis. As rapid growth & pigmentation is possible, so is confusion with melanoma. The 'dimple sign' is characteristic for dermatofibromas, where lateral compression results in central dimpling inwards. Treatment is conservative, but if in doubt of the diagnosis, excision biopsy is preferable.

Q: What is a furuncle & carbuncle?

Furuncles & carbuncles may affect any hair-bearing skin e.g. face, axilla & groin. They may be tender to palpation but have distinct differences as follows:

Terminology	Explanation
Furuncle	Perifollicular bacterial infection by *Staphylococcus aureus*. This results in a small, pus-containing swelling or 'boil'. As pus accumulates there is enlargement & punctum development. When the punctum bursts, the furuncle discharges spontaneously.
Carbuncle	A carbuncle is a cluster of furuncles that merge to form a larger lesion. They are often located at the back of the neck & are more common in diabetic patients. If present, investigation of blood glucose should be undertaken. Treatment may initially be conservative, however antibiotics may help. Good diabetic control will help to prevent further lesions in these patients. Large resistant lesions should be treated by surgical incision & drainage.

Q: What is a keratoacanthoma?

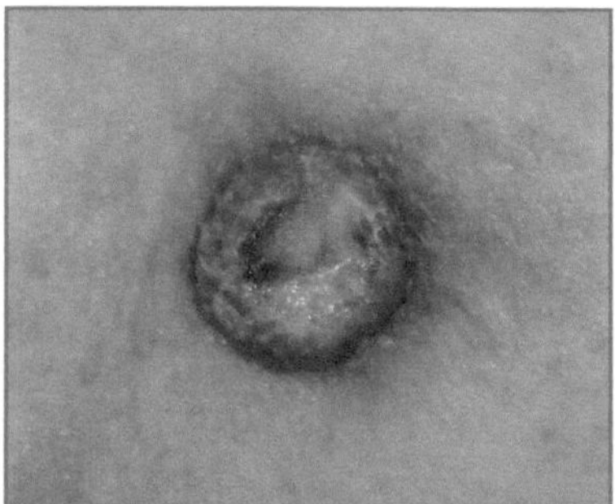

Fig 1.4: Keratoacanthoma.

A benign overgrowth of hair follicles, with a central keratin plug. Some consider this a type of self-limiting SCC. Keratoacanthomas may resemble some forms of BCC, SCC & melanoma, however spontaneously regress, leaving a depressed scar. Small biopsies will not be of diagnostic assistance, so an accurate history is important. They enlarge in weeks, remain static for 2–3 months & then resolve. The total cycle is 4–6 months.

Q: What are the treatment options for a keratoacanthoma?

Treatment	Examples
Conservative	**Monitoring** needs to be frequent due to the possibility of malignancy. This is very intense on outpatient clinics.
Surgical	**Treatment is usually by excision biopsy** as it is difficult to differentiate between a keratoacanthoma & SCC. This provides enough tissue for an accurate histological diagnosis.

Q: What is a naevus?

A benign proliferation of the normal constituent cells of the skin. Naevi may be classified as follows:

Classification	Example	Explanation
MELANOCYTIC	**Congenital**	Present at birth, often protuberant, hairy & pigmented (light brown-black). Often >1cm in diameter. There is a small risk of developing malignant melanoma (<5%).
	Junctional	Fig 1.5: Junctional naevus. Flat, round / oval pigmented macules that are often multiple. Lesions vary in size (typically 2–10mm) & colour (light–dark brown).
	Intradermal	Dome-shaped, flesh-coloured papules. Often seen on the face / neck.
	Compound	Pigmented nodules that appear warty / hairy & have variable pigmentation. They are usually <1cm in diameter.
	Blue	Usually solitary & named due to blue colour.
	Becker's	Pigmented, hairy naevus, commonly on the back / shoulder.
	Dysplastic	Irregular shape & pigmentation, with a high risk of malignant change.
VASCULAR	**Port Wine Stain**	Irregular red / purple macule, often affecting 1 side of the face.
	Salmon Patch	The most common vascular naevus, affecting almost 50% of neonates. Patches on the face often disappear, however posterior neck patches (stork marks) often persist.
	Strawberry Naevus	Also known as a capillary haemangioma, this usually develops during the 1st few weeks of life, reaching maximum size by 1 year. It is recognisable as a fleshy, red naevus that may affect the skin anywhere. Most regress spontaneously by the age of 8 years, leaving an area of atrophy.
EPIDERMAL	**Warty Naevus**	These may be present at birth or may develop during childhood. They are linear, pigmented, warty lesions that may grow to several centimetres in length. Recurrence is common after surgical excision.
CONNECTIVE TISSUE	**Shagreen Patches**	Rare soft, yellow, connective tissue naevus, associated with tuberose sclerosis, often found in the lumbar / sacral region.

Q: What is seborrhoeic keratosis?

A benign overgrowth of the basal cell layer of the epidermis. The following 3 features apply:

1. **Hyperkeratosis:** Thickening of the keratin layer.
2. **Acanthosis:** Thickening of the prickle cell layer.
3. **Hyperplasia:** Increased division of variably pigmented basaloid cells.

Q: What are the clinical features of seborrhoeic keratosis & how would you treat it?

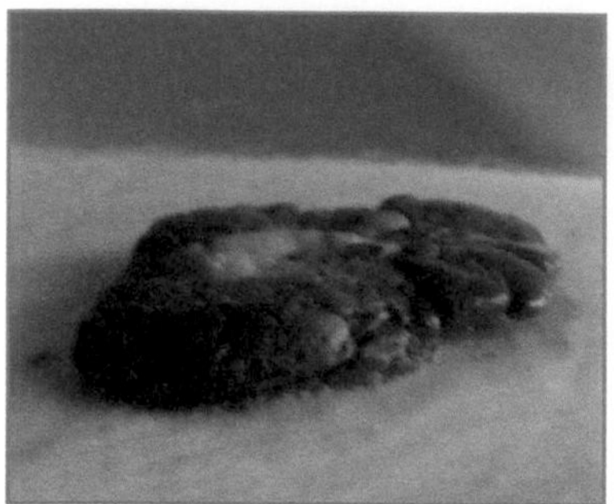

Fig 1.6: Seborrheoic keratosis.

Often seen on the face & trunk as variably pigmented lesions with a 'stuck on skin' warty appearance. They may be numerous & may scratch off easily & bleed. It is this & the pigmentation that causes concern, but they are benign. Patients may present with discomfort & irritation if they catch on clothing. Treatment is usually conservative & surgical treatment options include curettage, cryotherapy & cautery.

Q: What is a neurofibroma?

A benign hamartoma of peripheral nerve schwann cells. They may been seen as soft & fleshy pedunculated lesions of the skin. Altered sensation, pain & compressive symptoms may be present e.g. intra-abdominal neurofibromas may result in bowel obstruction & impingement on the spinal column may cause scoliosis or bone cysts. Treatment is usually conservative & surgical excision is possible.

Q: What is neurofibromatosis?

Neurofibromatosis represents 2 similar conditions, both inherited as autosomal dominant, classified into types I & II as follows:

Neurofibromatosis	Condition	Features
TYPE I	**Von Recklinghausen's Disease**	• ≥6 café-au-lait spots ≥0.5cm in diameter. • Multiple cutaneous neurofibromas that may be very large & can undergo sarcomatous change. • Increased risk of meningioma, acoustic neuroma & optic nerve glioma. • Kyphosis & tibial bowing may also occur.
TYPE II	**Bilateral Acoustic Neurofibromatosis**	These are more central than type I. Neurofibromas & café-au-lait spots are therefore not hallmark features, although may be present. Features include: • Bilateral acoustic neurofibromas. • Intracranial meningiomas. • Cranial nerve schwannomas.

Q: What is a papilloma?

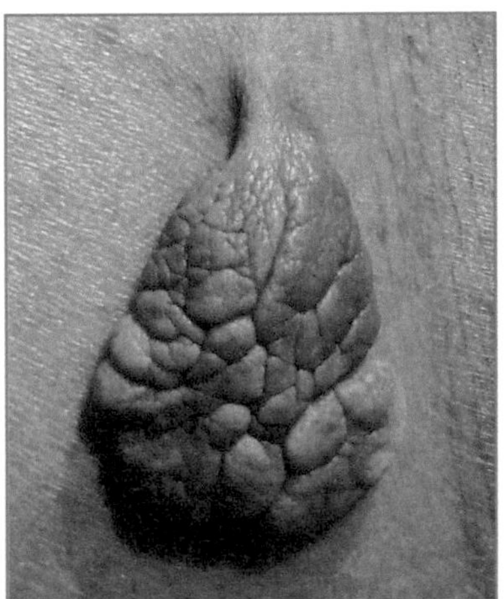

Fig 1.7: Large pedunculated papilloma.

A benign overgrowth of all skin layers, with a central vascularised core. Papillomas are fleshy, may vary in size & are also known as 'skin tags'. They may occur anywhere but are often seen on the face & neck. Treatment is by surgical excision.

Q: What is a pyogenic granuloma?

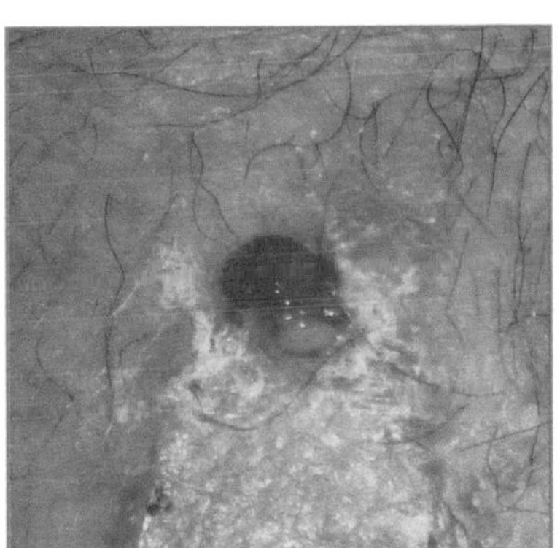

Fig 1.8: Pyogenic granuloma.

Unlike the name suggests, this is an acquired capillary haemangioma. Pyogenic granulomas are associated with a history of trauma. They present as soft raised lesions with a colour range from light red to deep purple. They may be painful & can bleed either spontaneously or with little trauma. They are best excised as this fixes the problem of bleeding & ensures tissue for histological diagnosis. **Note: Do not miss the amelanotic melanoma that looks like a pyogenic granuloma, especially if subungal.**

Q: What is a sebaceous (epidermoid) cyst?

An abnormal membrane-lined sac, composed of epithelial cells, containing a caseous substance with a 'cheesy odour'. This substance is comprised of:

- Fibrous tissue
- Fluid
- Keratin

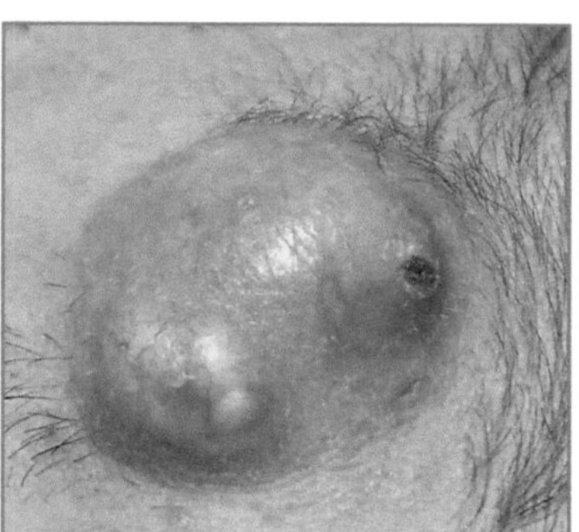

Fig 1.9: Sebaceous cyst.

Sebaceous cysts originate in the subcutaneous tissues so often seem fixed to skin. They may be of variable size with a central punctum. Discharge, ulceration & infection (abscess) may occur. Treatment is conservative unless symptomatic when surgical excision is indicated.

Q: What is a lipoma?

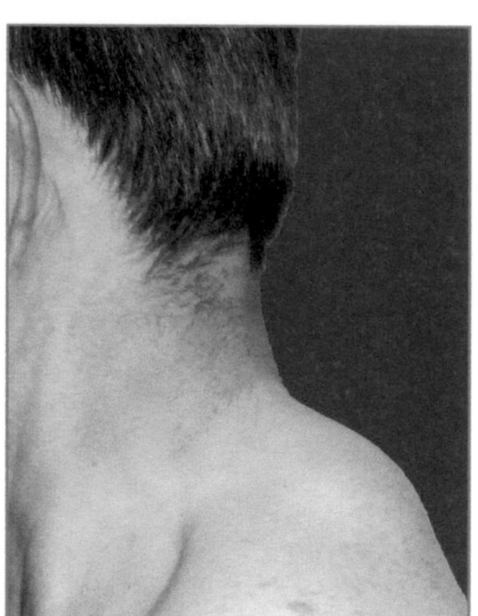

Fig 1.10: Large lipoma of the posterior neck / upper back.

A benign tumour of mature fat cells. Commonly seen on the neck & trunk & may become quite large. They originate in the fat layer, so are neither fixed to skin nor to underlying structures. They are freely mobile & it may be possible to demonstrate the 'slip sign' as the lump 'slips away' on palpation. Treatment is either conservative or surgical e.g. liposuction & excision biopsy. Liposuction leaves less scarring, but is associated with a higher recurrence.

Ulcers

Q: What is an ulcer?

A breakdown in all layers of an epithelial surface.

Q: What are the causes & 'edge features' of ulcers?

Classification	Notes	Edge
Traumatic	Ill fitting shoes / pressure sores.	Sloping
Venous (Fig 1.1)	Due to deep venous insufficiency & venous hypertension. Commonly seen over the malleoli.	Sloping
Infective	May be primary or secondary to infection of colonised chronic ulcers by e.g. Staphylococcus / Streptococcus	Sloping
Arterial	Painful. Often associated with peripheral arterial disease, particularly at pressure points e.g. between toes, plantar surface of foot, heel, metatarsal heads. May also be related to embolism or vasculitis.	Punched-Out
Neuropathic	Painless. Causes of neuropathy include diabetes, chronic alcohol abuse, leprosy or syphilis.	Punched-Out
Neoplastic	May be primary / secondary.	• Everted e.g. SCC / Marjolin's Ulcer • Rolled e.g. BCC

Q: What are the treatment options for ulcers?

- Treatment is of the underlying cause & complications.
- General strategies include:

Conservative	Medical	Surgical
Dressings	Antibiotics (if infective)	Ligation & Stripping (varicose veins)
Foot Elevation	Diabetic Control	Surgical Excision (neoplastic)
Orthopaedic Foot Wear		Skin Graft
Compression Stockings	**Note: 4 x layer compression bandaging of venous ulcers may be contraindicated in concurrent peripheral arterial disease e.g. ankle-brachial pressure index <0.8.**	

CHAPTER 2
HEAD & NECK

JA Joseph
BH Miranda
M Keene

CHAPTER CONTENTS

Thyroid Examination

Thyroid Status Examination

Neck Lump Examination

Parotid Gland Examination

Submandibular Gland Examination

OSCE Questions

- Thyroid Embryology
- Goitre and Thyroid Cancer
- Head & Neck Lumps
- Head & Neck Lymph Nodes
- Neck Dissection
- Parotid Gland
- Tonsillitis
- Epistaxis

THYROID EXAMINATION

START: Patient sitting on chair, with shirt unbuttoned / off.

Ask the patient to point out the lump if it is not clearly visible.

Inspect from FRONT, BACK, SIDES & ABOVE as follows:

INSPECTION	Interpretation
Lump	Goitre (Fig 2.1) & thyroglossal duct cysts are in the anterior triangle usually within 2cm of the midline.
6 x S's	Describe lump site, size, shape, symmetry, overlying skin & associated scars. **Note: The goitre may be butterfly shaped & symmetrical about the midline.**
Distended Veins	Distended neck veins imply SVC obstruction.
Swallow Water	Ask the patient to look up & swallow water. Goitres will move up.
Protrude Tongue	Ask the patient to look up & protrude tongue. Thyroglossal duct cysts will move up.

Ask about pain.

To prevent causing distress, explain to the patient that you will be feeling from behind.

Examine each side, accentuating the lobe by gently pressing the contralateral lobe towards the midline.

Examine the good side first.

Feel for temperature changes with the back of your hand.

PALPATION	Interpretation
SEC FFP TR	Palpate lump surface, edge, consistency, fixity to skin & underlying structures, fluctuance, pulsatility & expansility, transilluminability & reducibility. **Note: The goitre surface may be smooth or nodular.**
Feel Below Lump	Inability to get below the lump suggests retrosternal extension.
Swallow Water	Ask the patient to look up & swallow water. Goitres will move up.
Protrude Tongue	Ask the patient to look up & protrude tongue. Thyroglossal duct cysts will move up.
Trachea	Check for deviation.
Lymphadenopathy	Submental, submandibular, pre-auricular, post-auricular, occipital, posterior cervical, anterior cervical, pre-tracheal & supraclavicular.

PERCUSSION	Interpretation
Sternum	Percuss down sternum, checking for a dull-resonant interface. This suggests retrosternal goitre extension.

AUSCULTATION	Interpretation
Lump	Thyroid bruit in Graves' Disease.

COMPLETION	Interpretation
Thyroid Status	*See later.*
Vocal Fold Check	Refer to ENT specialist for FNE.

FINISH:

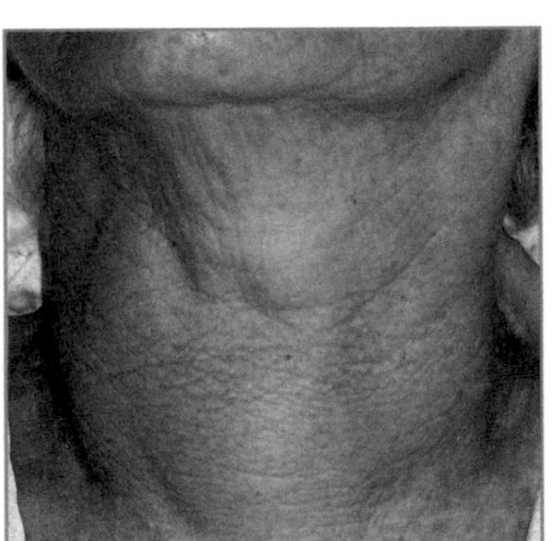

Fig 2.1: Goitre.

This is a large bilateral thyroid goitre. The right lobe is clearly visible & more enlarged than the left.

THYROID STATUS EXAMINATION

START: Patient sitting on chair, with shirt unbuttoned / off.

Inspect from FRONT, BACK & SIDES as follows:

General Appearance	Hyperthyroid	Hypothyroid
Demeanour	Restless	Docile
Hair	Normal	Brittle, Dry & Thin
Face	Wasting	Myxoedema Facies
Neck	Thyroid Swelling & Scars	Thyroid Swelling & Scars
Trunk	Weight Loss	Weight Gain

Hands	Hyperthyroid	Hypothyroid
Fingertips	Acropachy (Fig 2.2)	Normal
Palpation	Warm & Sweaty	Cold, Dry, Rough & Inelastic Skin
Paraesthesia	Usually Not Present	Carpal Tunnel Syndrome
Tremor	Present	Absent
Radial Pulse	Tachycardic / Irregular	Bradycardic

Eyes	Hyperthyroid	Hypothyroid
Lid Retraction	Present in Graves' Disease	Absent
Exophthalmos	Present in Graves' Disease	Absent
Lid Lag	Present in Graves' Disease	Absent
Sunken Eyes	Absent	Present
Periorbital Puffiness	Absent	Present
Loss of Outer Third of Eyebrow	Absent	Present

Shins	Hyperthyroid	Hypothyroid
Pretibial Myxoedema	Present in Graves' Disease	Absent

To test ankle reflexes position the patient with one knee on a chair & foot hanging over the edge.

Reflexes	Hyperthyroid	Hypothyroid
Ankle Reflex	Normal / Brisk	Slow Relaxing

To complete, perform a thyroid lump examination & ask questions relating to thyroid status as follows:

Question	Hyperthyroid	Hypothyroid
Mood Change	Anxiety	Depression
Appetite Change	Increased	Decreased
Body Temperature	Always Hot	Always Cold
Weight Change	Decreased	Increased
Hand Sensation	Usually Unaltered	Carpal Tunnel Syndrome
Heart Beat	Tachycardia & AF	Bradycardia
Bowel Habit	Diarrhoea	Constipation
Period	Menorrhagia	Oligomenorrhoea
Medication	Carbimazole & Propanolol	Levothyroxine
Operations / Radiotherapy	Total thyroidectomy is the commonest cause of hypothyroidism.	
Voice Change	Pressure of goitre on recurrent laryngeal nerve.	
Breathing Difficulty Lying Down	Pressure of goitre on trachea. This may also cause stridor.	
Swallowing Difficulty	Pressure of goitre on oesophagus causing dysphagia.	
Anaemia / DM / Pigmentation	Associated autoimmune disease.	

FINISH:

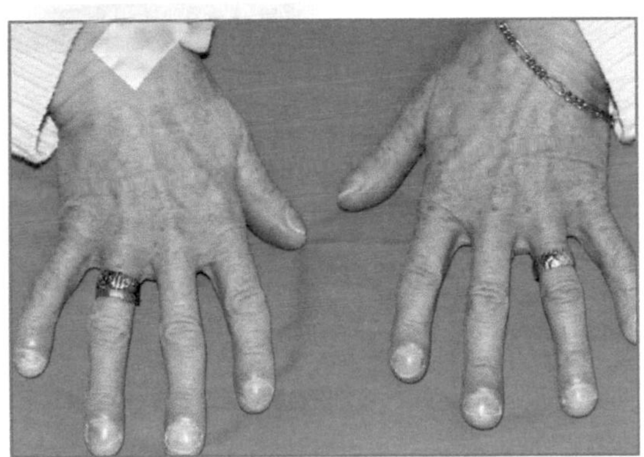

Fig 2.2: Digital Clubbing.

Digital clubbing associated with Grave's disease is known as thyroid acropachy.

NECK LUMP EXAMINATION

START: Patient sitting on chair, with shirt unbuttoned / off.

Ask the patient to point out the lump if it is not clearly visible.

Inspect from FRONT, BACK, SIDES & ABOVE as follows:

INSPECTION	Interpretation
General Appearance	*See thyroid status.*
6 x S's	Describe lump site, size, shape, symmetry, overlying skin & associated scars.
Distended Veins	Distended neck veins imply SVC obstruction.

If the lump is confined to the anterior triangle, test for thyroid swellings by asking patient to look up & swallow water, then look up & protrude tongue. If the lump moves up on swallowing or with tongue protrusion, continue palpation as for thyroid examination.

If the lump is confined to the posterior triangle, continue neck lump palpation as follows:

Ask about pain.

To prevent causing distress, explain to the patient that you will be feeling from behind.

Examine both sides of the neck, starting with the good side.

Feel for temperature changes with the back of your hand.

PALPATION	Interpretation
SEC FFP TR	Palpate lump surface, edge, consistency, fixity to skin & underlying structures, fluctuance, pulsatility & expansility, transilluminability & reducibility.
Neck Regions	Do not forget to palpate the remaining neck regions as there may be another lump.
Lymphadenopathy	Submental, submandibular, pre-auricular, post-auricular, occipital, posterior cervical, anterior cervical, pre-tracheal & supraclavicular.

AUSCULTATION	Interpretation
Lump	Bruit e.g. carotid / subclavian artery aneurysm.

The following examinations must be undertaken for completion if a neck lump is identified:

COMPLETION	Interpretation
ENT	Full ENT examination – refer to specialist for FNE.
Scalp & Face	Metastasis.
Axilla & Groin	Lymphadenopathy.
Breast	Metastasis.
Abdomen	Metastasis.

FINISH:

PAROTID GLAND EXAMINATION

START: Patient sitting on chair, with shirt unbuttoned / off.

Ask the patient to point out the lump if it is not clearly visible.

Inspect from FRONT, BACK, SIDES & ABOVE as follows:

INSPECTION	Interpretation
6 x S's	Describe lump site, size, shape, symmetry, overlying skin & associated scars (Fig 2.3).
Parotid Fistula	Previous operation.
Other Lumps	Do not forget to look at the contralateral side for bilateral parotid lumps. Look for possible lymphadenopathy.
Facial Nerve (VII)	Look for facial asymmetry, particularly looking at the nasolabial fold. Test muscles of facial expression 'raise eyebrows, shut eyes against resistance, blow out cheeks, show teeth, tense & flare neck muscles'. Facial nerve involvement suggests malignancy.
Oral Cavity	Using a pen torch, look for inflammation, pus & stones. Inspect the opening of **Stensen's Duct** in the buccal vestibule at the level of the maxillary 2nd molar.

Ask about pain.

To prevent causing distress, explain to the patient that you will be feeling from behind.

Examine both sides, starting with the good side.

Feel for temperature changes with the back of your hand.

PALPATION	Interpretation
SEC FFP TR	Palpate lump surface, edge, consistency, fixity to skin & underlying structures, fluctuance, pulsatility & expansility, transilluminability & reducibility. **Note: Asking the patient to clench their teeth will contract masseter, hence accentuating some parotid lumps & assisting in assessing fixity.**
Lymphadenopathy	Submental, submandibular, pre-auricular, post-auricular, occipital, posterior cervical, anterior cervical, pre-tracheal & supraclavicular.
Stensen's Duct	Palpate the opening of Stensen's Duct with the patient's mouth open. Try to milk the duct of any pus that may be present.
Bimanual	Use gloves, feeling for calculi & deep lobe tumours.

COMPLETION	Interpretation
Contralateral Side	Do not forget to examine the other side.
Chorda Tympani	Ask about change in taste sensation.
ENT	Full ENT examination – consider referral to specialist.

FINISH:

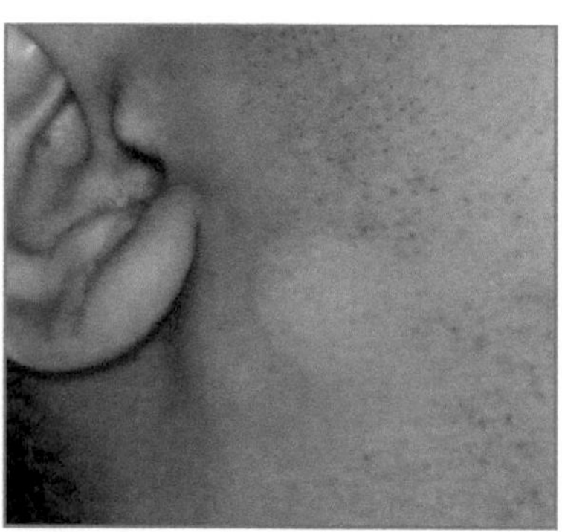

Fig 2.3: Right parotid pleomorphic adenoma.

SUBMANDIBULAR GLAND EXAMINATION

START: Patient sitting on chair, with shirt unbuttoned / off.

Ask the patient to point out the lump if it is not clearly visible.

Inspect from FRONT, BACK, SIDES & ABOVE as follows:

INSPECTION	Interpretation
6 x S's	Describe lump site, size, shape, symmetry, overlying skin & associated scars.
Other Lumps	Do not forget to look at the contralateral side for bilateral submandibular lumps. Look for possible lymphadenopathy.
Oral Cavity	Using a pen torch, look for inflammation, pus & stones. Inspect the opening of **Wharton's Duct** either side of the lingual frenulum.
Marginal Mandibular Nerve	Damage due to malignant infiltration / previous surgery results in an inability to depress the angle of the mouth. Facial asymmetry may also be seen here.
Hypoglossal Nerve (XII)	Damage due to malignant infiltration / previous surgery results in tongue deviation towards the side of the lesion with tongue protrusion.

Ask about pain.

To prevent causing distress, explain to the patient that you will be feeling from behind.

Examine both sides, starting with the good side.

Feel for temperature changes with the back of your hand.

PALPATION	Interpretation
SEC FFP TR	Palpate lump surface, edge, consistency, fixity to skin & underlying structures, fluctuance, pulsatility & expansility, transilluminability & reducibility.
Lymphadenopathy	Submental, submandibular, pre-auricular, post-auricular, occipital, posterior cervical, anterior cervical, pre-tracheal & supraclavicular.
Wharton's Duct	Palpate the opening of Wharton's Duct with the patient's mouth open. Try to milk the duct of any pus that may be present.
Bimanual	Use gloves, feeling for calculi & tumours.
Lingual Nerve	Damage due to malignant infiltration / previous surgery results in decreased touch sensation to the anterior two thirds of the tongue.

COMPLETION	Interpretation
Contralateral Side	Do not forget to examine the other side.
ENT	Full ENT examination – consider referral to specialist.

FINISH:

OSCE QUESTIONS

Thyroid Embryology

Q: What do you know about the embryology of the thyroid gland?

- 1st endocrine organ to develop.
- Development begins gestation day 24.
- Development begins between the 1st & 2nd pharyngeal pouches at the foramen caecum.
- Develops as a proliferation of endodermal cells on the pharyngeal floor, sited between the tuberculum impar & copula.
- Descent is via a pathway outlined by the thyroglossal duct (Fig 2.4).
- By gestation week 10, the thyroid gland lies with its isthmus over tracheal rings 2–4.
- The inferior parathyroid glands & thymus are derived from pharyngeal pouch 3.
- The superior parathyroid glands are derived from pharyngeal pouch 4.

Q: What are the clinical implications of disorders of thyroid gland embryology?

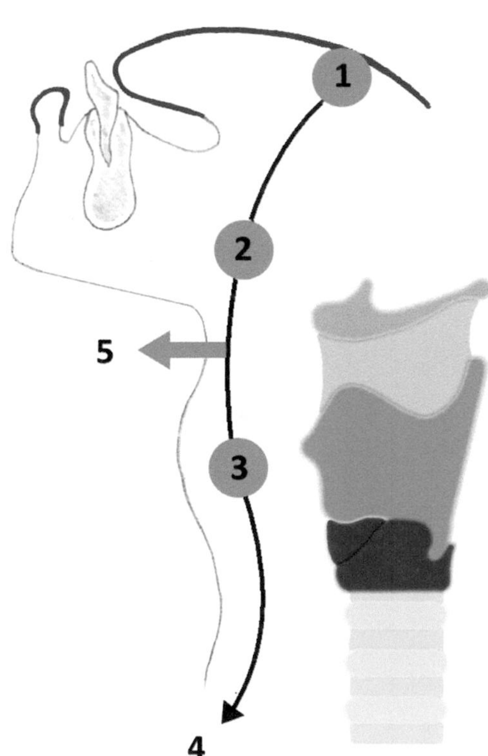

Clinical implications of thyroid gland embryology are due to the abnormalities of the normal pathway of descent & embryological development. Most of these disorders therefore lie along the pathway of the thyroglossal duct e.g. ectopic thyroid / retrostenal goitre.

Fig 2.4: Disorders of thyroid gland embryology.

1. **Lingual Thyroid:** Lump at the foramen caecum causing speech difficulty / dysphagia. Treatment is by surgical excision.
2. **Suprahyoid Thyroglossal Cyst:** *See later.*
3. **Infrahyoid Thyroglossal Cyst:** *See later.*
4. **Retrosternal Goitre:** *See above.*
5. **Thyroglossal Fistula:** Rarely congenital. Commonly due to infection / surgery. Treatment is by surgical excision.

Goitre & Thyroid Cancer

Q: How would you investigate a thyroid lump?

After taking a **full history** & performing a **thorough clinical examination**, I would consider the following tests:

Investigations	Notes
Blood Tests	FBC, U&E, LFT, CRP, TFT, Ca & Clotting.
USS & FNA	USS defines dimensions of tumour, if it is solitary / multinodular / solitary nodule / cyst. Cytology from FNA can reveal diagnosis.
Core Biopsy	Useful particularly if FNA is inconclusive.
CT / MRI	Defines complex anatomy, retrosternal extension, airway deviation or compression & oesophageal compression.
Radioisotope Scan	Identifies whether a nodule is ***'hot & functioning'*** (takes up isotope) or **'cold & non-functioning'** (no isotope uptake). Hot nodules are rarely malignant.

Q: How would you categorise the causes of thyroid swellings?

Goitre	Cause	Notes
NODULAR	**True Solitary Nodule**	50% have a true solitary nodule. Of these: 80% are adenomas. 10% are cysts, fibrosis or thyroiditis. 10% are cancer.
DIFFUSE	**Multinodular Goitre**	50% have a large nodule as part of a multinodular goitre.
	Physiological	Due to increased demand e.g. pregnancy.
	Dietary Iodine Deficiency	Rare but endemic to high altitude areas e.g. Alps & Himalayas.
	Dietary Goitrous Agents	Uncooked cabbage & turnips, calcium or fluoride in drinking water, various drugs.
	Graves' Disease	Patient is hyperthyroid & displays signs of Graves' Disease.
	Hashimoto's Thyroiditis	Autoimmune goitre & hypothyroid state.
	De Quervain's Thyroiditis	Self limiting & viral.
	Hereditary Errors of Thyroid Metabolism	Very rare autosomal recessive inborn errors of metabolism (8 types). They cause failure to respond to TSH or failure of T3 & T4 synthesis & release.
	Other	Lymphoma & amyloid.
	Congenital Absence or Atrophy of the Thyroid	If untreated leads to cretinism. Rarely associated with Pendred's Syndrome (congenital hypothyroidism & high tone deafness).

Q: What are the treatment options for benign thyroid swelling?

Classification	Treatment	Notes
CONSERVATIVE	**Remove Goitrogens e.g. Cabbage**	Reduce Thyroid Goitre.
MEDICAL	**Carbimazole**	If Hyperthyroid.
	Propylthiouracil	If Hyperthyroid.
	β-Blocker e.g. Propanolol	Symptomatic Relief of Hyperthyroidism.
	Thyroxine	If Hypothyroid.
SURGICAL	**Lobectomy** **Total Thyroidectomy**	**Indications:** • Diagnostic • Resolution of Compressive Symptoms e.g. Dysphagia, Dyspnoea & Dysphonia • Thyrotoxicosis Refractory to Medical Treatment e.g. Graves' Disease • Cosmetic

Q: What are the common thyroid cancers?

Thyroid Cancer	%	Notes
Papillary Adenocarcinoma	70	Common in children. 90% have lymphatic metastases at presentation.
Follicular Carcinoma	20	Common around 50 years. Blood-borne spread.
Medullary Carcinoma	5	Parafollicular C cell origin. Produce calcitonin. 90% are sporadic, 10% are MEN related.
Anaplastic Carcinoma	<5%	Common in older patients.
Lymphoma	<5%	Core biopsy best for diagnosis. Treat with DXT & chemotherapy.

Q: What are the treatment options for malignant thyroid disease, diagnosed following FNAC?

Diagnosis	Treatment	Notes
Papillary Adenocarcinoma	Thyroid Hormone Suppression Hemithyroidectomy.	Some centres advocate this when tumour <1cm (T1 stage).
	Radio-Iodine Ablation. Total Thyroidectomy & Level VI Neck Dissection.	For tumours greater than 1cm (T2–4 stage).
Follicular Adenocarcinoma	Hemithyroidectomy.	Usually performed in the 1st instance as it is difficult to distinguish adenoma (benign) from adenocarcinoma (malignant) on FNAC.
	Radio-Iodine Ablation. Total Thyroidectomy.	Completion thyroidectomy & level VI neck dissection performed if histology shows malignancy, followed by radio-iodine ablation.
Medullary Thyroid Cancer	Total Thyroidectomy.	Completion thyroidectomy & level VI neck dissection, with removal of any other suspicious lymph nodes. Requires lifelong calcitonin (tumour marker) follow up.
Anaplastic Carcinoma	Surgical Debulking, DXT & Doxorubicin.	Survival is around 1 year only.

Q: Do you know any inherited syndromes causing tumours of the endocrine system?

Multiple endocrine neoplasia (MEN), is inherited in an autosomal dominant manner & may be classified by type as follows:

Type	Notes
MEN I	**Memory: 3 x P's** • **P**ancreatic Islet Cell Tumour • **P**ituitary Adenoma • **P**rimary Hyperparathyroidism
MEN IIa	**Memory: 3 x C's** • **C**atecholamines (Phaeochromocytoma) • **C**alcitonin (Thyroid Medullary Carcinoma) • **C**alcium (Primary Hyperparathyroidism)
MEN IIb	Same features as MEN IIa without parathyroid involvement. Also: • Marfanoid Habitus • Multiple Neuromas

Head & Neck Lumps

Q: Can you list some causes of neck lumps in the regions labelled 1–6?

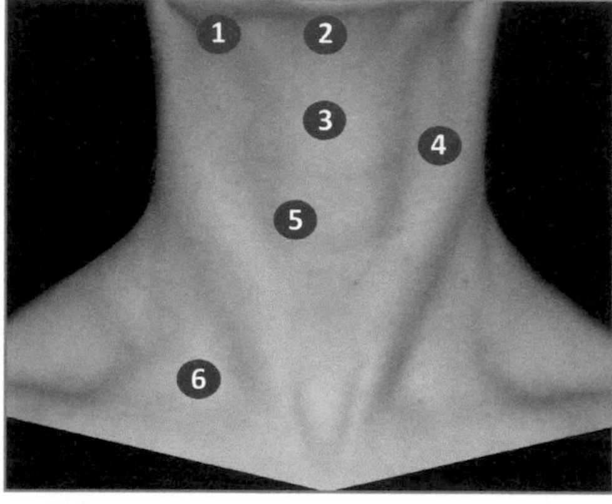

1. Submandibular Gland Swelling
   Chemodactoma (expansile)
2. Submental Gland Swelling
   Dermoid Cyst
3. Thyroglossal Cyst
4. Branchial Cyst
5. Thyroid Nodule
6. Cystic Hygroma
   Tip of Cervical Rib
   Subclavian Artery Aneurysm (expansile)

Q: What investigations would you order for a neck lump & in what order?

Investigations	Notes
Bloods	FBC, U+E, LFT, CRP & Clotting CMV, EBV, *Toxoplasma & Bartonella.*
USS & FNA	Will provide diagnosis if squamous cell carcinoma, infective or inflammatory.
CT / MRI	Helps locate primary tumour. Neck, chest, abdomen & pelvis images assist staging.
Lymph Node Biopsy	Required when FNA inconclusive e.g. Lymphoma.

Q. What are the causes of neck lumps?

These include the causes for any lump (*see lumps 'n' bumps chapter*) & those specific to the neck as follows:

Classification	Location	Cause	Notes
CONGENITAL	Anterior Triangle	**Congenital Dermoid Cyst**	Affects children & young adults. Commonly on lateral & medial aspect of eyebrow & anywhere in the midline at sites of embryological fusion.

Classification	Location	Cause	Notes
		Thyroglossal Duct Cyst	Cyst lying along the tract of the obliterated thyroglossal duct. 90% in midline. Most occur in childhood. Excised by Sistrunk's Procedure. This removes the cyst, middle third of hyoid & any thyroglossal duct remnants.
		Sternomastoid Tumour	Caused by birth trauma. Head turned away & tilted toward affected side. Painful to turn head. Treated with surgical tenotomy.
	Posterior Triangle	**Cystic Hygroma**	Type of lymphangioma. Occur in lower neck. Treat with surgical excision.
ACQUIRED	Anterior Triangle	**Implantation Dermal Cyst**	In areas subjected to repeated trauma e.g. fingers. Seen rarely in the neck. Due to forcible implantation of skin subcutaneously.
		Branchial Cyst	Thought to arise from elements of squamous epithelium in a lymph node. Usually in young adults. 60% are in males. Lie deep to anterior border of SCM at junction of upper & mid third in anterior triangle.
		Thyroid Lump	*See above*
		Parotid Tumour	*See below*
		Submandibular Swelling	*See below*
		Chemodectoma	Nearly always benign. There are many types e.g. carotid body tumour. This arises from the carotid bulb & may be pulastile. Rare except in high altitude areas e.g. Mexico City.
		Pharyngeal Pouch	Caused by herniation of pharyngeal mucosa (pulsion diverticulum) through weak point in its muscular coat (Killian's Dehiscence) between thyopharyngeus above & cricopharyngeus below (2 muscles of inferior constrictor). Most commonly in elderly. Occasional cystic swelling in low anterior neck. Causes regurgitation of undigested food. Diagnosed with barium swallow. (Fig 2.5) If troublesome treated with endoscopic pouch stapling.

Classification	Location	Cause	Notes
		Carotid Artery Aneurysm	Expansile mass. Caused by atheroma, infection or trauma. Resect if causing TIAs.
		Laryngocoele	Laryngeal air sac from increased intra-laryngeal pressure e.g. glassblowers.
	Posterior Triangle	**Cervical Rib**	Palpable bony swelling in supraclavicular fossa. Cause of thoracic outlet syndrome.
		Lipoma	Commonly in posterior triangle & overlying trapezius.
		Subclavian Artery Aneurysm	Sometimes palpable in supraclavicular fossa. Often due to thoracic outlet syndrome.
	All Regions	**Lymphadenopathy**	*See later* (Fig 2.6).

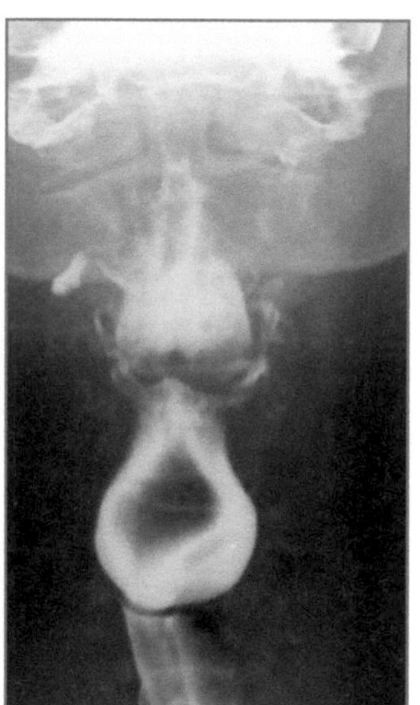

Fig 2.5: Pharyngeal pouch.

Barium swallow delineating a pharyngeal pouch.

Head & Neck Lymph Nodes

Q: What lymph nodes should be routinely examined in the head & neck?

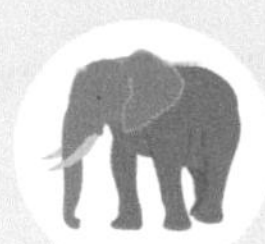

Memory: Examine for head & neck lymphadenopathy systematically, standig behind the patient. You can use the order presented (Fig 2.6). Your hands should move in a sweeping motion without going backwards & forwards. Feel & compare both sides. This looks more 'slick' to the examiner.

Nodes	Notes
Submental	Underneath chin & anterior third of mandible.
Submandibular	Underneath mandible body.
Pre-Auricular	Anterior to pinna of ear, over mandible ramus.
Post-Auricular	Behind the ear over the mastoid bone.
Anterior (Deep) Cervical Chain	Follows the course of the IJV in the neck. Can be palpated along the anterior border of sternocleidomastoid.
Posterior (Superficial) Cervical Chain	Within the posterior triangle along trapezius.
Occipital	Over the occipital bone at the back of the skull.
Supraclavicular	Within the posterior triangle along the posterior-superior border of the clavicle.
Pre-Tracheal	In midline overlying the trachea.

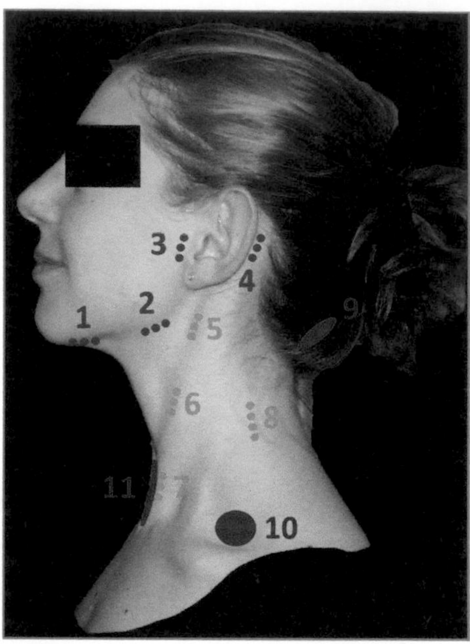

Fig 2.6: Head & neck lymphadenopathy.

Key	Nodes	Level
1	Submental	I
2	Submandibular	I
3	Pre-auricular	-
4	Post-auricular	-
5	Anterior / Deep Cervical (Upper)	II
6	Anterior / Deep Cervical (Middle)	III
7	Anterior / Deep Cervical (Lower)	IV
8	Posterior / Superficial Cervical	V
9	Occipital	-
10	Supraclavicular	VI
11	Pre-Tracheal	VI

Note: Current practice in ENT is to describe cervical lymphadenopathy in terms of levels (I–VI) as follows:

Level	Notes
I	Submental & submandibular nodes within the digastric triangle.
II	Upper anterior / deep cervical chain nodes around the upper third of the IJV, where it is crossed anteriorly by the spinal accessory nerve. This level extends from the skull base in the region of the jugular foramen to the carotid bifurcation (Fig 2.7).
III	Mid anterior / deep cervical nodes around the middle third of the IJV, from the carotid bifurcation to the cricothyroid notch.
IV	Lower anterior / deep cervical nodes around the lower third of the IJV, from the cricothyroid notch to the clavicle.
V	Posterior triangle nodes between the posterior border of SCM & anterior border of trapezius. This also includes the supraclavicular nodes.
VI	Anterior compartment of the neck adjacent to the thyroid & trachea.

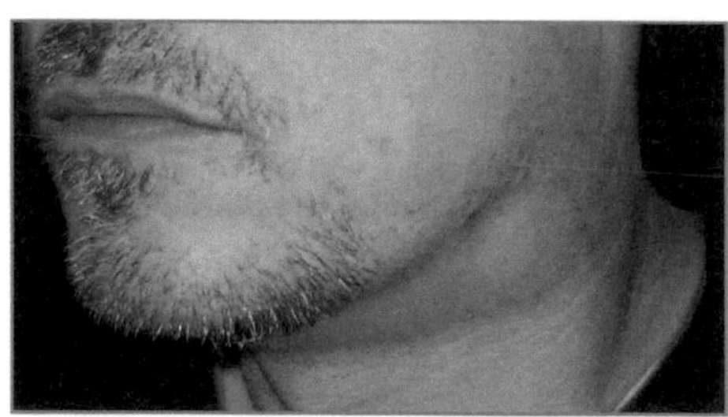

Fig 2.7: Level II lymphadenopathy.

Neck Dissection

Q: What do you understand about neck dissection?

There are several types of neck dissection described for head & neck tumours:

Dissection Type	Notes
Radical	*Removal of:* • Level I-V lymph nodes. • Accessory nerve. • Sternocleidomastoid muscle (SCM). • Internal jugular vein (IJV).
Modified Radical	*Removal of:* • Level I-V nodes... Then subclassified as: • **Type 1:** Preserve accessory nerve. • **Type 2:** Preserve accessory nerve & SCM. • **Type 3:** Preserve accessory nerve, SCM & IJV.
Extended Radical	Radical dissection with removal of paratracheal & mediastinal lymph nodes & parotid gland.
Selective	Depends on lymph node level taken.

Parotid Gland

Q: What tests would you order to investigate a parotid lump & in what order?

Investigations	Notes
Bloods	FBC, U+E, LFT, CRP, Ca, clotting, rheumatoid factor, autoantibody screen (Sjögren's Syndrome).
USS & FNA	Will reveal stones. Delineates tumour & can provide cytological diagnosis.
Sialogram	Shows anatomy of ductal system & any stones present. Can be therapeutic intervention (crush stone or grasp & remove).
MRI	If concerned about complex anatomy or deep lobe involvement.

Q: What are the causes of diffuse parotid swelling?

Cause	Notes
Infective	Causing acute / chronic parotitis & may be: **Viral:** Coxsackie, Echovirus Mumps, & HIV. **Bacterial:** Actinomycosis, *Staphylococcus* & TB.
Inflammatory	**Sjögren's Syndrome:** An autoimmune disease often associated with rheumatoid arthritis. Symptoms include parotidomegaly, xerostomia & keratoconjunctivitis sicca. **Mikulicz's Syndrome:** Similar to Sjögren's Syndrome, characterised however by salivary & lacrimal gland enlargement. Must have an associated underlying cause e.g. TB / Sarcoid.
Drugs	Alcohol, OCP, Thiouracil, Phenylbutazone & Isoprenaline.
Metabolic	Bulimia, Cirrhosis, Cushing's Disease, Diabetes, Gout & Myxoedema.
Sialectasis	Progressive destruction of the parotid gland occurs, accompanied by duct stenosis & cyst formation. May be either congenital or acquired through epithelial debris / calculi.
Pseudo-Parotidomegaly	The following may mimic parotid swelling: • Cyst • Lipoma • Preauricular Lymphadenopathy • Facial Nerve (VII) Neuroma • Hypertrophic Masseter • Winged Mandible • Mandible Tumour • Branchial Cyst • Dental Cyst

Q: What are the causes of a parotid gland tumour?

Classification	Example	Notes
BENIGN	**Pleomorphic Adenoma** (Fig 2.2)	Commonest of all salivary gland neoplasms. 80% of parotid tumours. Peak incidence in 5th decade.
	Warthin's Tumour (papillary cystadenoma)	Also known as a papillary cystadenoma. Peaks around the 7th decade & is 7 times more prevalent in males.
	Monomorphic Adenoma	Group of rare tumours. Most common is basal cell adenoma. Presents in 6th decade.
	Lymphangioma	Rare congenital hamartoma. Usually present before age 2. Removed for cosmetic reasons.
	Haemangioma	Most common in children.
	Neurofibroma	Rare in parotid. Nerve sheath tumour. Originates from facial nerve (VII).
VARIABLE MALIGNANCY	**Mucoepidermoid Carcinoma**	Most prevalent salivary neoplasm in children. This can act like a benign or malignant tumour.
	Acinic Cell Carcinoma	This can act like a benign or malignant tumour.
MALIGNANT	**Adenoid Cystic Carcinoma**	The most prevalent malignant parotid tumour. Peaks around the 6th decade.
	Adenocarcinoma	Develops within secretory ducts. Local & distant metastases present in 33% of presentations.
	Undifferentiated Carcinoma	Uncommon, high-grade cancer. Tumour size is an important prognostic indicator.
	Lymphoma	Commonly affects elderly men. Biopsy is indicated as treatment includes chemotherapy / radiotherapy.

Q: How would you classify the clinical features & causes of facial nerve palsy?

Classification	Clinical Features	Causes
UPPER MOTOR NEURON	• Hemifacial palsy. • Able to raise eybrow due to bilateral innervation of frontalis & orbucularis oculi.	**Cerebrovascular Accident:** Suspect in the elderly & those at risk of ischaemic or haemorrhagic events.
		Multiple Sclerosis
		Meningitis
		Acoustic Neuroma
		Glioma

Classification	Clinical Features	Causes
LOWER MOTOR NEURON (Fig 2.8)	• Hemifacial palsy. • Unable to raise eyebrow.	**(55%) Bell's Palsy:** Unknown aetiology so is a diagnosis of exclusion. Theoretical viral or ischaemic cause. Treat with high dose oral steroids & acyclovir for 7 days if <72 hours. 85% fully recovered after 3 months.
		(19%) Trauma: Iatrogenic e.g. parotidectomy, Blunt or Penetrating.
		(7%) Ramsay Hunt Syndrome: Herpes zoster viral infection resulting in shingles of the facial nerve (VII). Characteristic vesicles are seen in the ear canal.
		(6%) Tumour: Either of the facial nerve (VII) e.g. schwannoma, due to invasion e.g. malignant parotid tumour or extrinsic pressure e.g. vestibular nerve schwannoma.
		Infection: Acute or chronic suppurative otitis media. Malignant otitis externa.
MIXED	Upper & lower motor neuron lesion signs.	Causes are rare e.g. sarcoid, myasthenia gravis, Guillain-Barré syndrome & drugs.

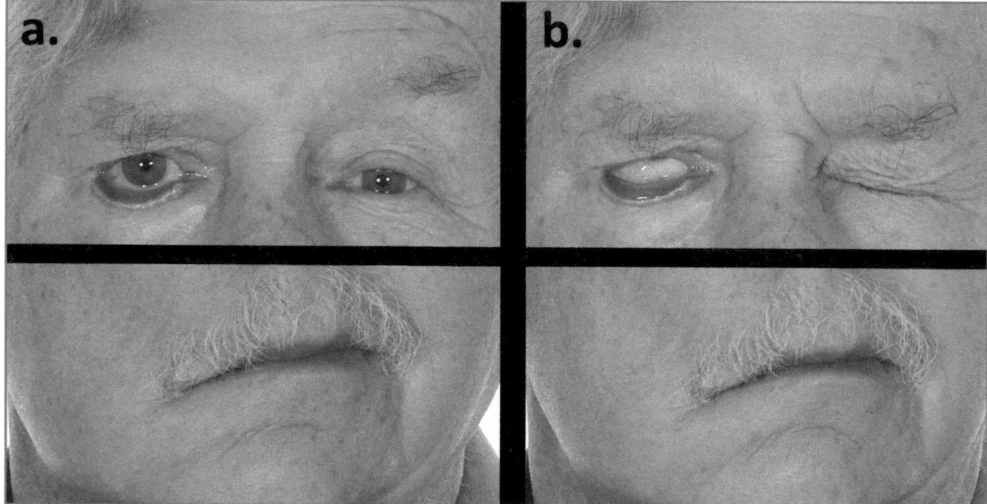

Fig 2.8: Right facial nerve lower motor neuron involvement.

(a) This patient has a right-sided facial droop, with loss of the right forehead furrow. (b) When the patient is asked to shut his eyes, the right eye does not close & deviates superiorly (Bell's Reflex).

Q: What is Sjögren's Syndrome?

This is an autoimmune disease, 90% of which is seen in women around 50 years of age. Periductal lymphocytes in multiple organs is characteristic at histology. 50% of cases have salivary gland involvement. Lymphoma affects 1 in 6 patients. The syndrome may be classified as follows:

- **Primary:** Keratoconjunctivitis Sicca & Xerostomia
  No Connective Tissue Disorder Association
- **Secondary:** Connective Tissue Disorder Association:
  - Rheumatoid Arthritis
  - Systemic Lupus Erythematosus
  - Scleroderma

Q: What specific investigations would assist your diagnosis of Sjögren's Syndrome?

Investigation	Notes
Schirmer's Test	Hyposecretion: the lacrimal glands may be tested by inserting a special strip of filter paper under the lower eyelid. Hyposecretion is confirmed by wetting of the filter paper <5mm in 5 minutes (normal 15mm).
Autoantibodies	Rheumatoid factor, anti-Ro & anti-La.
Sublabial Biopsy	Salivary gland histology.

Q: What are the treatment options for a patient with Sjögren's Syndrome?

Conservative	Medical	Surgical
Meticulous Oral Hygiene	Artificial Tears	Lacrimal Punctum Diathermy
Antibacterial Mouth Wash	Steroids	
Monitoring for Lymphoma	Immunosuppressants	

Tonsillitis

Q: What are the causes of acute tonsillitis?

Viral	Bacterial
Influenza	β-Haemolytic *Streptococcus*
Parainfluenza	*Streptococcus pneumoniae*
Adenovirus	*Haemophilus influenzae*
Enterovirus	Anaerobic Organisms
Rhinovirus	
Epstein Barr Virus (EBV)	

Q: What are the clinical features of tonsillitis (Fig 2.9)?

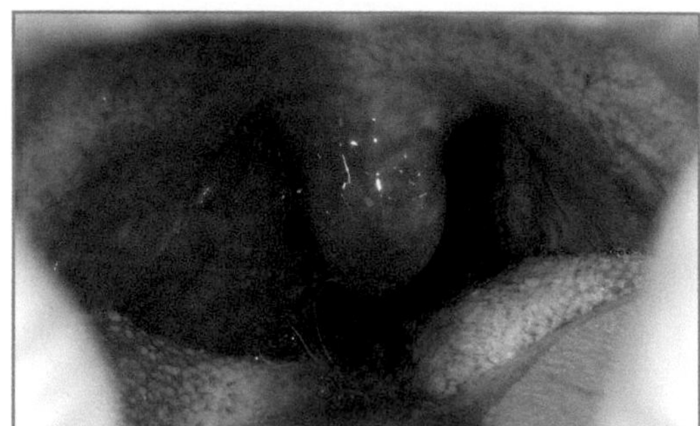

Fig 2.9: Acute right-sided tonsillitis.

The patient has an enlarged, erythematous right tonsil.

Clinical Features	Notes
Pyrexia, Malaise & Headache	Often prodromal for 24 hours.
Hyperaemic Tonsils, Pus & Debris in Crypts	Clinically diagnostic for infective tonsillitis.
Sore Throat	The predominant symptom.
Muffled Voice	Due to generalised oedema. A 'hot potato voice' may be present, so-called due to sounding like the voice of a person trying to speak with hot potatoes in their mouth! The significance is a possible **Quinsy**.
Neck Pain	There may be associated cervical lymphadenopathy.
Odynophagia	Pain on swallowing.
Trismus	Difficulty opening mouth.
Tender Jugulodigastric Lymphadenopathy	Enlarged regional nodes in upper neck (level I and II).
Quinsy	Peritonsillar abscess seen as a collection of pus around the tonsil. Requires drainage under local anaesthetic.
Respiratory Obstruction	Severe swelling causing obstruction & respiratory distress.

Q: What investigations would you consider for a patient with suspected tonsillitis?

After taking a **full history** & performing a **thorough clinical examination**, I would order the following tests:

Investigation	Example	Explanation
BLOOD TESTS	**Paul-Bunnell / Monospot Test**	Detects EBV in glandular fever (infectious mononucleosis).
	FBC	Expect raised WBC. Neutrophilia if bacterial cause. Lymphocytosis if viral cause.
	CRP	Acute phase reactant.
MICROBIOLOGY	**Throat Swab / MC+S**	Useful if empirical treatment not working.
	Blood Cultures	Detect bacteraemia.

Q: What treatment would you implement for a patient with confirmed tonsillitis?

Medical	
Analgesia & Antipyretics	Reduce pain & temperatures.
Penicillin	Aerobic cover. Erythromycin may be used if the patient is penicillin allergic. **Note: Avoid amoxicillin as it causes a generalised rash in patients with glandular fever.**
Metronidazole	Anaerobic cover.
Dexamethasone	Reduces inflammation & particularly useful in severe cases.
Hospital Admission	
IV Antibiotics	In extreme cases, when the patient is unable to tolerate fluids orally, the patient is not safe for discharge & requires hospital admission for IV treatment.
IV Fluids	
IV Analgesia	
Surgical	
Tonsillectomy	For recurrent cases (>5 episodes in each of 2 consecutive years).

Q: What are the complications of tonsillitis?

Complication	Notes
Respiratory Obstruction	Severe swelling causing obstruction & respiratory distress.
Quinsy	Peritonsillar abscess seen as a collection of pus around the tonsil. Requires drainage under local anaesthetic.
Parapharyngeal / Retropharyngeal Abscess	May require drainage under general anaesthetic.
Acute Otitis Media	Due to tracking infection along eustachian tube.
Recurrent Acute Tonsillitis	Tonsillectomy is indicated with >5 episodes in each of 2 consecutive years.

Epistaxis

Q: What is epistaxis?

Acute haemorrhage from the nostril, nasal cavity of nasopharynx. This may either be anterior (90% of cases) or posterior. Anterior bleeds mostly arise from Little's area, which is richly vascularised (Kiesselbach's plexus). Posterior bleeds mostly arise from Woodruff's plexus.

Q: What are the causes of epistaxis?

These may be classified as local / systemic as follows:

Local	Systemic
Nose Picking	Hypertension
Trauma (direct / barotrauma)	Blood Dyscrasias
Infection (upper respiratory tract)	Drugs (aspirin / warfarin / heparin)
Allergy (sinusitis / rhinitis)	Alcohol Abuse
Substance Abuse (cocaine)	Liver Failure
Tumors	Haematological Anaemias
Iatrogenic (nasal cannulae / nasogastric tube)	

Q: What are the clinical features of epistaxis?

- Overt bleeding from the nasal cavity.
- Posterior bleeding from the nasopharynx may be visualised in the oropharynx.
- Massive epistaxis may mimic haemoptysis / haematemesis.

Q: What are the treatment options for expistaxis?

This is an emergency and must be managed in the context of either the acute life support (ALS) or acute traumatic life support (ATLS) protocols, addressing ABCs (**A**irway, **B**reathing, **C**irculation). The underlying cause must also be addressed. Specific treatment options include:

Conservative	Medical	Interventional / Surgical
Direct Pressure (20 Minutes)	(IV) Fluid Resuscitation	Embolisation*
Nasal / Post-Nasal Packing	Adrenaline Spray	Ligation*
Epistaxis Balloon	Cautery	***Arteries involved include the sphenopalatine, posterior ethmoidal, maxillary.**
Stop Aspirin / Warfarin / Heparin	Antibiotics (especially after packing)	

SECTION A2: TRUNK & THORAX

CHAPTER 3
BREAST

BH Miranda
DT Sharpe

CHAPTER CONTENTS

(also see book 1 oncology & operative surgery chapters)

Breast Examination

OSCE Questions

- Fibroadenoma
- Excessive Breast Development
- Cyclical Nodularity & Mastalgia
- Breast Cyst
- Duct Ectasia
- Periductal Mastitis
- Epithelial Hyperplasia
- Fat Necrosis
- Breast Tumours
- Paget's Disease of the Nipple
- Management of Breast Disease

BREAST EXAMINATION

START: Patient exposed from the waist upwards, lying at 45°.

Maintain the patient's dignity using e.g. bed sheet.

Chaperone is vital.

When asked to examine the breasts, remember to systematically examine as follows:

1. Lumps should be considered as any other lump & should be addressed first.
2. Features of breast disease should be considered next.
3. The above points should be considered both with the patient's hands behind their head (to accentuate lumps, asymmetry & tethering) & pushing against their hips (to accentuate lumps attached to the pectoralis muscle). It is additionally possible to inspect the breasts with the patient leaning forward over the side of the bed (to accentuate abnormalities in large breasts).
4. Once all the above points are addressed for the 'good' breast first, remember afterwards to compare with the 'diseased' breast i.e. inspect for lumps & breast features of the good breast, then the diseased breast; then palpate for lumps & breast features of the good breast, then the diseased breast.

If you are asked to examine a breast lump that you are unable to identify, you may wish to ask the patient if they have noticed any lumps anywhere.

INSPECTION	Interpretation
6 x S's	Describe lump site, size, shape, symmetry, overlying skin & associated scars (*see lumps 'n' bumps chapter)*.
Fungation	Comment on presence of fungating carcinoma. It is important to **check the inframammary fold** that may hide a fungating carcinoma & other breast signs.
Asymmetry	Carcinoma may be present in the higher breast (Fig 3.1).
Tethering	Due to infiltration of the ligaments of Astley-Cooper.
Peau D'Orange	Due to micro-oedema.
Lymphoedema	May indicate lymphatic infiltration by carcinoma, or previous surgery with lymph node removal.
Nipple Signs	**Memory: Remember the 6 x D's of nipple disease:** • Paget's **D**isease (Fig 3.2) • **D**ischarge • **D**epression • **D**eviation • **D**isplacement • **D**estruction

Ask about pain.

Remember to examine the good breast first, then the diseased breast, according to the system described above.

Check for temperature changes, using the back of your hand.

PALPATION	Interpretation
SEC FFP TR	Palpate lump surface, edge, consistency, fixity to skin & underlying structures, fluctuance, pulsatility & expansility, transilluminability & reducibility.
Breast	Palpate the breast using the palmar surfaces of the index, middle & ring fingers of both hands in succession, sweeping down the clock face positions of the good breast first, then the diseased breast. Remember to thoroughly examine each breast with the patient's hands behind their head, then pressing against their waist. **Note: Most carcinomas present in the upper, outer quadrant of the breast.**
Inframammary Fold	This is often forgotten & must be specifically palpated.
Axillary Tail of Spence	This is often forgotten & must be specifically palpated.
Nipple Discharge	Explain to the patient that it is important for you to check for a discharge by gently squeezing the nipple & gain permission to do so.
Axillary Lymphadenopathy	Palpate for axillary lymphadenopathy, facing the patient, by supporting their arm with your corresponding arm. You will then be able to use your free hand to palpate for lymphadenopathy i.e. support the patient's right arm with your right arm, then examine the right axilla with your left hand. It may be easier to examine the left axilla with the patient sitting on the edge of the bed. Remember to examine the anterior, posterior, medial & lateral walls in addition to the apex.
Supraclavicular Lymphadenopathy	This is often forgotten & must be specifically palpated.

COMPLETION	Interpretation
Surgical Complications	Consider the nerves that may have been damaged in a post-mastectomy patient e.g. long thoracic nerve of Bell (winging of the scapula) & intercostobrachial nerve (loss of sensation in the distribution of T2).
Respiratory Exam	May indicate metastases.
Abdominal Exam	May indicate metastases.
Spinal Exam	Spinal tenderness in particular may indicate metastases.
Encourage Self Exam	Encourage the patient to regularly monitor their breasts, using a simple examination technique in front of the mirror.
Triple Assessment	If a lump is suspected / detected, complete triple assessment (*see below*).

FINISH:

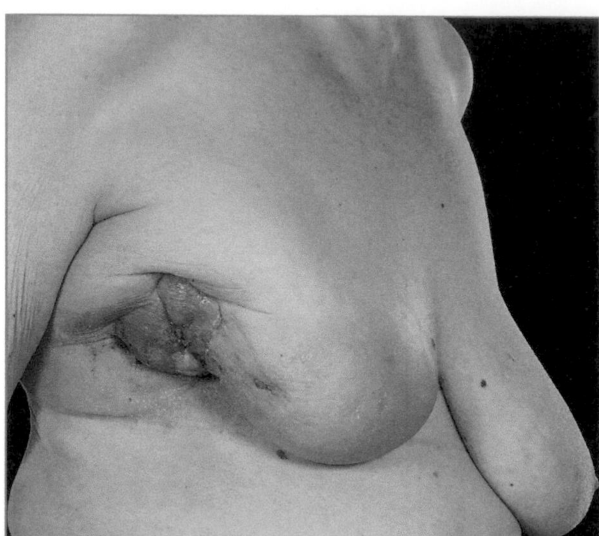

Fig 3.1: Carcinoma of the right breast & marked breast asymmetry, with the right breast lying higher than the left.

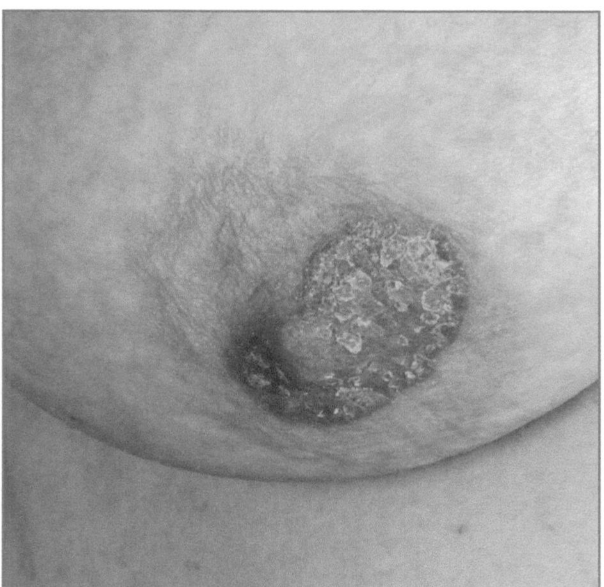

Fig 3.2: Paget's Disease of the nipple.

OSCE QUESTIONS

Q: How would you classify breast disease?

Breast disease may be classified as **benign** or **malignant**. The aetiology of benign breast disease may be classified as aberrations of normal development & involution (ANDI). ANDI was first introduced at an international breast conference in Cardiff & describes abnormal processes of development, involution & cyclical hormonal activity as follows:

Peak Age (years)	Process		Aberration
15–25	**Development**		Fibroadenoma & Excessive Breast Development
25–40	**Cyclical Hormonal**		Cyclical Nodularity & Mastalgia
35–55	**Involution**	*Lobular:*	Cysts
		Ductal:	Duct Ectasia & Periductal Mastitis
		Epithelial:	Hyperplasia & Fibrosis

Note: Malignancy is more prevalent in females over the age of 55 years.

Q: What is a fibroadenoma?

The most common benign neoplasm in females. It is a fibroepithelial tumor, composed of glandular tissue & stroma. The peak age of onset is 15–25 years. Clinically, it presents as a painless, smooth, firm & rubbery lump that is highly mobile. Approximately 10% will resolve spontaneously within 1 year.

Q: What is excessive breast development?

Excessive enlargement of the breast due to glandular & stromal proliferation. Minor degrees may be seen in infants due to the effect of maternal oestrogens. Females with excessive breast development may have a hormonal imbalance or hormone-secreting tumour. Males with excessive breast development have gynaecomastia. The causes of excessive breast development are classified as follows:

Classification	Cause
Physiological	Puberty & Pregnancy
Pathological	Hormone-Secreting Tumours, Hypogonadism & Liver Cirrhosis
Pharmacological	Cimetidine, Digoxin, Spironolactone & THC

Q: What are cyclical nodularity & mastalgia?

These affect pre-menopausal females & are hormone dependent. Cyclical breast changes occur, resulting in lumps (nodularity) & pain (mastalgia) related to the menstrual cycle. Treatment options may be classified as follows:

Conservative	Medical	Surgical
Reassurance	Evening Primrose Oil	Mastectomy (for treatment resistant severe mastalgia)
Firm Supporting Bra	Analgesia	
Evening Primrose Oil	Oral Contraceptive Pill	
	Danazol	
	Bromocriptin	
	Tamoxifen	

Q: What are breast cysts?

Breast cysts are fluid-filled, distended & involuted lobules. They present as smooth lumps that may be painful & have a peak age of onset of 35–55 years. Fine needle aspiration may relieve symptoms by drainage of cystic fluid that may then be analysed by microbiology & cytology.

Q: What is duct ectasia?

Duct ectasia is characterised by involution & dilation of the subareolar ducts. Clinical features may include nipple inversion, nipple discharge (may be blood stained), subareolar mass & mastalgia.

Q: What is periductal mastitis?

Periductal mastitis refers to inflammation, often with associated infection, of the subareolar ducts. It may present in a similar manner to duct ectasia, with a subareolar mass, pus discharge from the nipple & mastalgia. When bacterial infection is involved, broad spectrum antibiotics will almost always resolve the issue.

Q: What is epithelial hyperplasia?

Epithelial hyperplasia is characterised histologically by an increase in the number of epithelial lining cells of the terminal duct lobular unit. When atypical dysplasia is present, there is an increased risk of progression to carcinoma.

Q: What is fat necrosis?

Fat necrosis often occurs after trauma to the fatty breast tissue e.g. during breastfeeding or surgery. Inflammation, fibrosis & calcification may ensue. Clinically fat necrosis may be difficult to distinguish from carcinoma as it presents as a hard, irregular lump, sometimes tethered to skin or associated with axillary lymphadenopathy. Most cases resolve spontaneously.

Q: How would you classify breast tumours?

Tumours of the breast may be classified as benign, pre-malignant or malignant as follows:

Benign	Pre-Malignant / *in situ*	Malignant / Invasive
Fibroadenoma	Ductal Carcinoma *in situ*	Invasive Ductal Carcinoma (80% of invasive)
Intraductal Papilloma	Lobular Carcinoma *in situ*	Invasive Lobular Carcinoma (10% of invasive)
Lipoma		Invasive Medullary, Mucinous, Tubular & Papillary Carcinomas (10% of invasive)

Q: What is Paget's Disease of the nipple?

Paget's Disease of the nipple (Fig 3.2) is an eczematous nipple presentation that, when present, is almost always associated with underlying carcinoma. 2% of all carcinomas are associated with Paget's Disease. Clinical features include persistent nipple erythema, crusting, paraesthesia & pain.

Q: What investigations should be ordered to guide management of breast disease?

Investigations must be tailored towards the suspected underlying aetiology, however, employing the concept of **triple assessment** is vital:

Triple Assessment Stage	Interpretation
1. Clinical Examination	Clinical examination is the first part of triple assessment.
2. Imaging	Mammogram / USS
3. Tissue Sampling	FNAC / Core Biopsy / Open Biopsy

To assess metastasis, the following investigations are useful:

- **LFTs & Liver USS** (liver)
- **CXR** (chest)
- **Radioisotope Bone Scan** (bone)
- **CT Brain** (brain)

CHAPTER 4
ABDOMEN

BH Miranda
MJ Portou
MC Winslet

CHAPTER CONTENTS

Abdominal Examination

OSCE Questions

- Clubbing
- Upper Gastrointestinal
- Hepatobiliary
- Spleen
- Kidneys
- Lower Gastrointestinal
- Rectum and Anus
- Common Abdominal Scars

ABDOMINAL EXAMINATION

START: Patient lying flat & exposed to underwear ideally, to allow for hernia & PR examinations. This also allows for thorough examination e.g. the chest wall for spider naevi or gynaecomastia & both legs for oedema.

Use sheet covers appropriately, to maintain patient dignity.

INSPECTION	Interpretation
Moving Abdomen	No guarding. Guarding is the maintenance of a rigid abdomen, to reduce pain.
Cough	May reveal a hernia.
Head off Bed	Asking the patient to lift their head off the bed may reveal divarification of the rectus abdominis at the linea alba. This may also reveal a hernia.
Caput Medusa	Distended periumbilical veins *(later in chapter).*
Scars	Previous surgery.
HANDS:	
Hepatic Asterixis	A *'liver flap'* is often encephalopathy associated. It occurs due to delivery of toxins, usually metabolised by the liver, to the brain.
Leukonychia	Nail whitening due to hypoalbuminaemia.
Koilonychia	Nail spooning due to Fe deficiency.
Clubbing	*(later in chapter)*
Palmar Erythema	Localised vasodilation due to decreased oestrogen.
Dupuytren's Contracture	This may be idiopathic, familial, associated with chronic liver disease or Peyronie's Disease *(see hand chapter).*
WRIST / ARM:	
Excoriations	Pruritis.
Needle Marks	IVDU is associated with HBV & HCV transmission.
Tattoos	HBV & HCV transmission from tattoo needles.
Bruising	Clotting abnormality.
Pulse	Check Rate & Rhythm. Rate increases in acute pancreatitis, perforation & 3rd space fluid loss.
FACE:	
Pale Conjunctiva	Anaemia sign.
Yellow Sclera	Jaundice.
Corneal Arcus	May be congenital or associated with chronic cholestasis & hypercholesterolaemia. It may also develop inconsequentially after the age of 50.

Xanthelasma	Fleshy, yellow, subcutaneous deposits of cholesterol, often around the eyelids & eyes.
Kayser-Fleicher Rings	Copper deposits present in Wilson's Disease. **Note: These are only truly seen with the use of a slit lamp, so mention this!**
MOUTH:	
Glossitis	Vitamin B12 deficiency.
Angular Stomatitis	Fe & Vitamin B12 deficiency.
Aphthous Ulcers	Crohn's Disease, Behcet's Disease & HSV.
Pigmentation	**Peutz-Jegher's Syndrome** is an autosomal dominant condition associated with mucosal pigmentation & gastrointestinal hamartomatous polyps. Mucosal pigmentation is also seen in Addison's Disease.
Telangiectasia	**Osler-Weber-Rendu Syndrome** is an autosomal dominant condition associated with haemorrhagic telangiectasia of the mucous membranes e.g. oral & nasal, gastrointestinal tract & lungs. Epistaxis & gastrointestinal bleeding are common features.
NECK:	
Troisier's Sign	***The presence of a left supraclavicular lymph node, also known as Virchow's Node.*** Associated with gastrointestinal carcinomas, particularly gastric carcinoma.
CHEST:	
Gynaecomastia	Due to decreased oestrogen metabolism by damaged hepatocytes.
Spider Naevi	***Branched, dilated arterioles that blanch with pressure & refill from the centre outwards; >5 – abnormal.*** Due to decreased oestrogen metabolism.
Axillary Hair Loss	Due to decreased oestrogen metabolism.
ABDOMEN:	
6 x S's	Describe lump / mass site, size, shape, symmetry, overlying skin & associated scars (Fig 4.1).
Distension	**Memory:** **The 5 x F's of Abdominal Distension.** Fat Fluid Faeces Flatus Foetus
Visible Peristalsis	Kneel down & look across the abdomen for peristalsis due to bowel obstruction.
Aortic Pulsations	Kneel down & look across the abdomen for AAA pulsations.
Scars	Ensure you roll the patient to check for more posterior scars *(later in chapter)*.

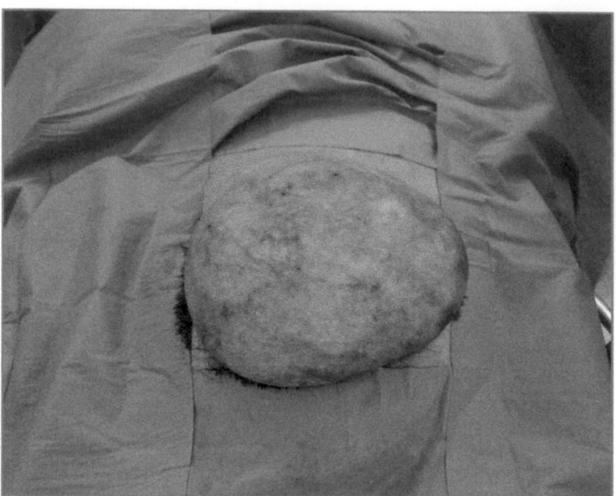

Fig 4.1: Large abdominal mass.

Ask about pain.

Look at the patient's face throughout the examination.

Warm your hands by rubbing them together & warn the patient that they may be cold.

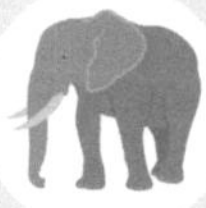

Memory: The 9 x regions of the abdomen: 1 x epigastric, 2 x hypochondrium, 1 x umbilical, 2 x lumbar, 1 x suprapubic & 2 x iliac (Fig 4.2).

PALPATION	Interpretation
9 Regions SOFT	Localising tenderness & superficial lumps / masses. **Guarding** may be palpated as the patient tenses their abdominal muscles to *'guard'* inflamed abdominal organs from pain upon pressure. Guarding may be classified as voluntary or involuntary as follows: • **Voluntary:** A conscious & deliberate contraction of anterior abdominal wall muscles to prevent deeper palpation. Relaxation occurs once pressure is released. • **Involuntary:** Reflex anterior abdominal wall muscle spasm caused by peritoneal inflammation which cannot be wilfully suppressed.
9 Regions DEEP	Localising deep lumps / masses.
SEC FFP TR	Palpate lump / mass surface, edge, consistency, fixity to skin & underlying structures, fluctuance, pulsatility & expansility, transilluminability & reducibility.
Liver	Use the radial border of your right index finger, thumb & fingers extended, to palpate from right iliac fossa to right hypochondrium. Describe the distance below the costal margin (cm).
Spleen	Use the tips of your right index, middle & ring fingers to palpate from right iliac fossa to left hypochondrium. Rolling the patient towards you may assist palpation. The spleen has a notch, you can't get above it, it enlarges to the right iliac fossa & is not ballotable.
Kidneys	Ballot the kidneys. Kidneys have no notch, you can get above them, they enlarge vertical-inferior & are ballotable.
Gall Bladder	Where the right border of rectus crosses the costal margin.
Abdominal Aortic Aneurysm	Palpate for expansility, with thumbs & fingers extended, running your index fingers parallel to the abdominal aorta. This is usually best localised above the umbilicus, just left of midline.

PERCUSSION	Interpretation
Liver	Delineate extension (cm) beyond the costal margin.
Spleen	Delineate extension (cm) beyond costal margin.
Ascites	Demonstrate **shifting dullness**. Start percussion from the umbilicus away from you. Demonstrate the resonant (air) to dull (fluid) interface at the flanks & leave your finger at that point. Roll the patient towards you & maintain that position for a few minutes, allowing gravity to drain peritoneal fluid. Continue percussion in the same direction, demonstrating that what once was dull, has now *'shifted'* to resonant! The presence of fluid may be further confirmed by demonstrating a **percussion thrill**.

AUSCULTATION	Interpretation
Bowel Sounds	Describe frequency & quality e.g. hyperdynamic & tinkling.
Hepatic Bruit	Hepatocellular carcinoma.
Aortic Bruit	AAA.
Renal Bruit	Renal artery stenosis.

COMPLETION	Interpretation
Lymphadenopathy	Check inguinal lymph nodes.
Hernial Orifices	Inguinal hernias.
External Genitalia	Full examination.
Digital Rectal Exam	Identify mass, blood or mucus.
Urine Dipstick	Glycosuria.
Fluid Chart	If available.
Stool Chart	If available.
Ankle Oedema	Hypoalbuminaemia *(see vascular chapter for other causes).*

FINISH:

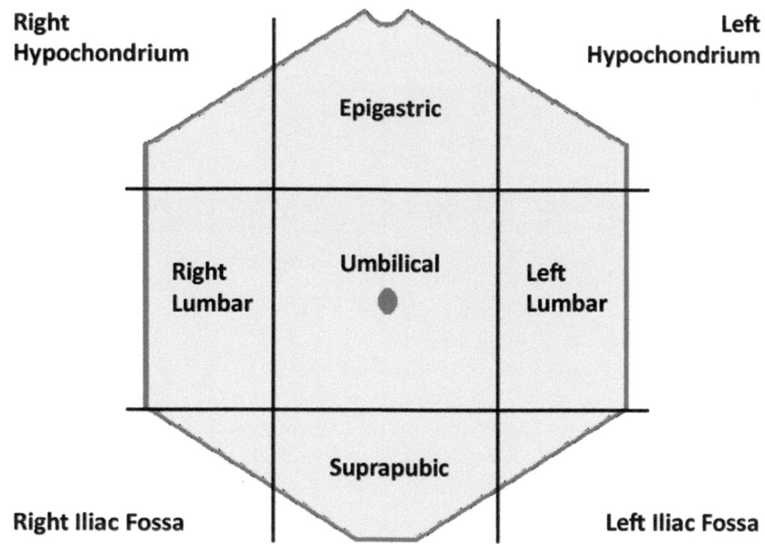

Fig 4.2: The 9 abdominal regions.

OSCE QUESTIONS

Clubbing

Q: What are the stages of clubbing (Fig 2.2)?

1. Congestion
2. Loss of Angulation
3. Increased AP Diameter
4. Drumsticking

Q: What are the causes of clubbing?

Clubbing may be idiopathic. Other causes are classified as follows:

Gastrointestinal	Respiratory
Cirrhosis	Bronchial Carcinoma
Inflammatory Bowel Disease	Chronic Suppurative e.g. Abscess, Bronchiectasis & Empyema
Malabsorption Diseases	Fibrosing Alveolitis
Lymphoma	Mesothelioma
Cardiovascular	**Rare**
Infective Endocarditis	Graves' Disease (thyroid acropachy)
Cyanotic Congenital Heart Disease	Familial

Upper Gastrointestinal

Q: What is dysphagia?

Difficulty swallowing.

Q: What are the causes of dysphagia?

These may be classified as oropharyngeal & oesophageal, or as follows:

Congenital		
Oesophageal Atresia		
Acquired		
LUMINAL	**INTRAMURAL**	**EXTRAMURAL**
Food Bolus	Achalasia*	Hilar Lymphadenopathy
Foreign Body	Carcinoma	Pharyngeal Pouch
Oesophageal Web	GORD	Retrosternal Goitre
Plummer-Vinson Sydrome*	Oesophagitis	Lung Carcinoma
	Oesophageal Dysmotility	
	Scleroderma	
	Stricture e.g. Radiation*	

NEUROLOGICAL	OTHER
Stroke	Stomatitis
Myasthenia Gravis	Glossitis
Motor Neurone Disease	Tonsillitis & Pharyngitis

* Associated with an increased risk of developing malignancy. Plummer-Vinson Syndrome is the presence of an oesophageal web, associated with Fe deficiency anaemia.

Q: What is odynophagia?

Pain on swallowing.

Q: Can you give a spot diagnosis for the 3 conditions depicted in the barium swallows below?

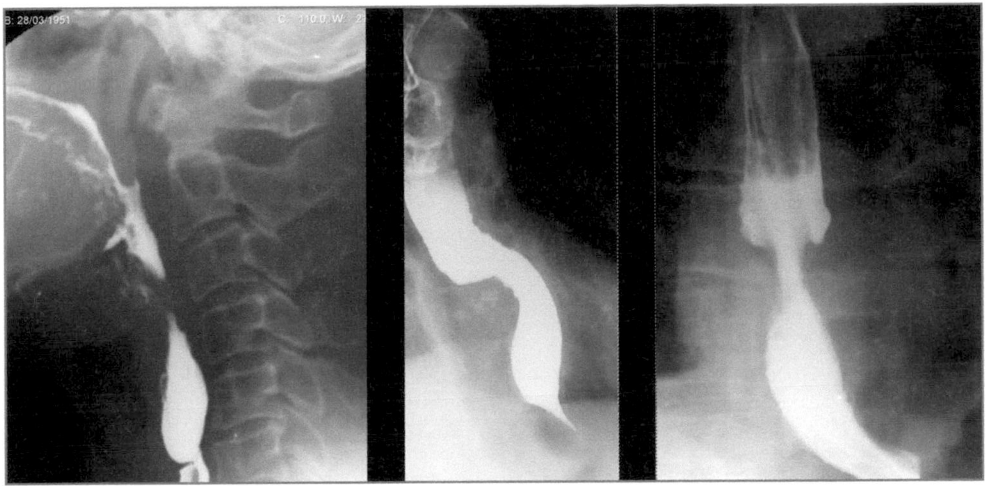

Fig 4.3: Barium swallows of patients with different causes of dysphagia.

Left = oesophageal web. Middle = achalasia (bird's beak / rat's tail sign). Right = oesophageal carcinoma (shouldered stricture)

Q: What are the causes of odynophagia?

Many causes of dysphagia also result in odynophagia. Below are some of the common causes:

Cause	Examples
Trauma	Pharyngeal Trauma, Radiation, Oesophageal Burn, Mallory-Weiss Syndrome & Ruptured Oesophagus
Foreign Body	Oropharyngeal & Oesophageal
Infection	Pharyngitis, Tonsillitis, Oesophagitis (HSV & Candida) & Abscess
GORD	Oesophagitis & Ulceration
Neoplasia	Pharyngeal, Laryngeal & Oesophageal Carcinoma
Motility	Achalasia & Oesophageal Dysmotility Syndromes
Neurological	Stroke, Myasthenia Gravis & Motor Neurone Disease
Other	Plummer-Vinson Syndrome, Pharyngeal Pouch & Scleroderma

Q: What are the causes of an epigastric mass?

Skin & Soft Tissue	Gastrointestinal	Vascular
Cyst	Epigastric Hernia	AAA
Lipoma	Gastric Carcinoma	Lymphadenopathy
Sarcoma	Pancreatic Carcinoma	
	Pancreatic Pseudocyst	

Hepatobiliary

Q: What are the causes of hepatomegaly?

Physiological	Alcohol Related
Riedel's Lobe	Cirrhosis
Hyperexpanded Chest	Fatty Liver
Infective	**Metabolic**
Hepatitis, EBV & CMV (virus)	Amyloid
TB & Abscess (bacteria)	Hereditary Haemochromatosis (HHC)
Malaria & Schistosomiasis (protozoa)	Wilson's Disease
Malignant	**Congestive**
Primary / Secondary	Right Heart Failure
Lymphoma	Tricuspid Regurgitation (pulsatile liver)
Leukaemia	Budd-Chiari Syndrome

Q: What are the most common causes of hepatomegaly in the UK?

Cause	Explanation
Malignancy	This may be primary or secondary & includes haematological malignancies e.g. CML.
Alcohol Related	Fatty Liver Disease & Alcoholic Hepatitis.
Infective	Viral e.g. HAV, HBV, HCV & EBV. Bacterial e.g. Liver Abscess. Parasitic e.g. Malaria (following foreign travel).

Q: What is Budd-Chiari Syndrome?

Budd-Chiari Syndrome is due to hepatic vein obstruction from e.g. thrombosis or carcinoma. The clinical picture includes upper abdominal pain, jaundice, hepatomegaly & ascites. LFTs are often deranged & progression to encephalopathy may occur.

Q: What are the causes of cirrhosis?

Congenital	**Cardiac**
HHC	Congestive Cardiac Failure (CCF)
Wilson's Disease	**Drugs**
α1-Antitrypsin Deficiency	Alcohol*
Autoimmune	**Infective**
Hepatitis	HBV / HCV*
Biliary	Schistosomiasis**
Primary Biliary Cirrhosis (PBC)	**Other**
Primary Sclerosing Cholangitis (PSC)	Sarcoid

* Common causes

** Important in Asia, Africa & South America

Q: What is portal hypertension & what are the causes?

Portal hypertension is defined as a portal vein pressure >10mmHg. Causes may be classified as pre-hepatic, hepatic or post hepatic as follows:

Pre-Hepatic	Hepatic	Post-Hepatic
Portal Vein Thrombosis	Cirrhosis	Budd-Chiari Syndrome
Splenic Vein Thrombosis	Sarcoid	Constrictive Pericarditis
Splenic Arteriovenous Fistula	Schistosomiasis	Right Heart Failure

Q: What are caput medusae?

Distended, engorged periumbilical veins, due to severe portal hypertension with porto-systemic shunting of blood through the umbilical veins.

Causes of distended umbilical veins may be:

1. Physiological
2. Portal hypertension leading to porto-systemic shunting
3. IVC obstruction

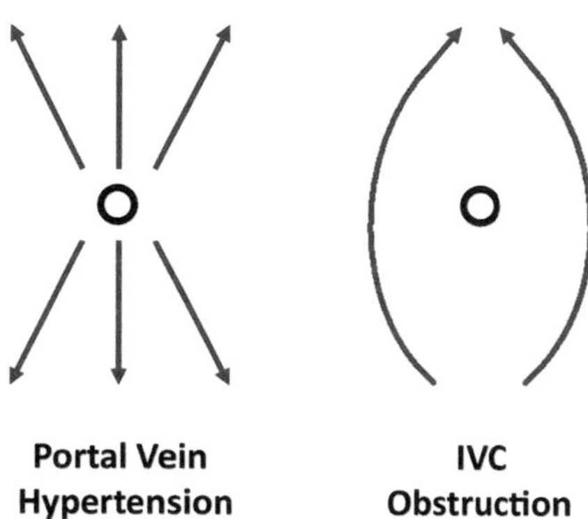

Fig 4.4: Diagram showing direction of blood flow with causes of umbilical vein distension.

Note direction of blood flow in diagram.

Q: What is ascites?

Fluid in the peritoneal cavity.

Q: What are the causes of ascites?

These may be classified as transudate or exudate as follows:

TRANSUDATE (Protein < 30g/L)	EXUDATE (Protein > 30g/L)
Cirrhosis	Inflammation e.g. Pancreatitis
Nephrotic Syndrome	Infection e.g. TB
CCF	Malignancy (Primary / Secondary)
Pericarditis	

Q: How would you investigate ascites?

Investigation	Examples		
Blood Tests	FBC, U&E, LFT, CRP & Coagulation.		
Diagnostic Paracentesis	Note appearance of fluid. Send for	MICROBIOLOGY:	MC&S
		CYTOLOGY:	Malignant Cells
		BIOCHEMISTRY:	Protein / Glucose / Amylase
Serum Ascites Albumin Gradient	Better clinical indicator than protein content alone. If the difference between the serum & ascites albumin concentrations is <1.1, an exudate is present. If >1.1, a transudate is present.		
USS	Diagnostic USS may be used to assess intra-abdominal organs & extent of ascites. It may also be used to guide drainage procedures.		
Doppler	May demonstrate portal vein flow, Budd-Chiari Syndrome & portal vein thrombosis.		
Abdominal CT	Further imaging of intra-abdominal organs.		

Q: What are the treatment options for ascites?

Classification	Treatment	Explanation
CONSERVATIVE	**Salt Restriction**	Assists production of urine to off-load fluid.
	Weight Monitoring	Quantifies diuresis. The weight loss goal is no more than 0.5kg/day for ascites alone. If patients have additional peripheral oedema, the weight loss goal is no more than 1kg/day.
	Water Restriction	If hyponatraemia is present.
MEDICAL	**Cause**	Treating the underlying cause will prevent progression of ascites.
	Diuretics	Spironolactone is the drug of choice. Otherwise a loop diuretic e.g. furosemide.
SURGICAL	**Paracentesis**	This may be diagnostic & therapeutic.
	TIPS	Transjugular intrahepatic portosystemic shunts, between the portal & hepatic veins, may be used in patients with advanced cirrhosis & recurrent ascites.
	LeVeen Peritoneovenous Shunt	Peritoneovenous shunts drain ascites directly into the venous circulation. They connect the peritoneal cavity to the SVC / IJV via a one-way valve to prevent back flow of blood. Short-term complications include fluid overload, long-term complications include shunt blockage, bacterial colonisation & infection.
	Liver Transplant	For end stage liver disease.

Q: What are the causes of gall bladder enlargement?

Causes may be classified according to the associated presence or absence of jaundice as follows:

Jaundiced	Not Jaundiced
Pancreas Carcinoma (Head)	Mucocoele
Cholangiocarcinoma	Empyema
	Gall Bladder Carcinoma
	Acute Cholecystitis

Note: Gallstones may cause chronic inflammation of the gallbladder. This results in fibrosis & thickening of the wall which does not become distended. Hence, painless jaundice in the presence of a palpable gallbladder is unlikely to be due to gallstone disease (the principle behind Courvoisier's Law).

Spleen

Q: What are the functions of the spleen?

Function	Explanation
Reticuloendothelial System	Filters & removes RBCs, WBCs & platelets.
Storage	Holds 35% of body platelet stores.
Immunological	The destruction, via phagocytosis, of encapsulated organisms e.g. *Haemophilus influenzae, Streptococcus pneumoniae* & *Neisseria meningitidis.*
Synthesis	Synthesises antibodies & opsonin (enhances phagocytosis).

Q: What are the causes of splenomegaly?

Haemolytic Anaemia	Neoplastic
Sickle Cell	Leukaemia e.g. Chronic Myeloid*
Thalassaemia	Myelofibrosis*
Elliptocytosis	Non Hodgkin's Lymphoma
Spherocytosis	Tumour (Primary / Secondary)

Infective	Splenic Vein Hypertension
Abscess, TB & Endocarditis (bacteria)	Cirrhosis
HIV, IM & Hepatitis (virus)	Budd-Chiari Syndrome
Malaria* & Schistosomiasis (protozoa)	Portal Vein Thrombosis
Hydatid Cyst (parasite)	**Other**
Inflammatory	Amyloid
Rheumatoid Arthritis	CCF
Sarcoid	Felty's Syndrome

* These are causes of massive splenomegaly.

Q: What is hypersplenism?

Hypersplenism is defined by the presence of the following:

1. Splenomegaly
2. Cytopaenia*
3. Normal or Hyperplastic Bone Marrow
4. Response to Splenectomy**

* Cytopaenia may take the form of anaemia, leukopaenia, thrombocytopaenia or pancytopaenia.

** Response to splenectomy implies that hypersplenism is a retrospective diagnosis.

Kidneys

Q: What are the causes of a kidney mass?

Congenital	Neoplastic
Simple Solitary Cyst	Adenoma
Polycystic Kidney Disease (PCKD)	Renal Cell Carcinoma
Horseshoe Kidney	Wilms' Tumour
Hypertrophic Single Kidney	2° Metastasis
Infective	**Vascular**
Abscess	Infarction
Hydatid Cyst	Renal Vein Thrombosis
TB	**Other**
Inflammatory	Amyloid
Sarcoid	Hydronephrosis

Q: What is PCKD?

Polycystic kidney disease is characterised by the presence of bilateral renal cysts. It is an important cause of renal failure & may be classified as infantile or adult, with the following characteristics:

Characteristics	Infantile	Adult
Genetics	Autosomal recessive.	Autosomal dominant.
Presenting Years	Commonly at birth / infancy (prenatal USS now picks this up *in utero*).	Commonly in adults (although may present at any time).
Presenting Symptoms	Renal mass & poor renal function.	Usually in 5th decade with declining renal function. Also mass, loin pain, haematuria & hypertension.
Associations	Hepatic fibrosis, leading to portal hypertension & splenomegaly.	40% have berry aneurysms with risk of subarachnoid haemorrhage.
Prognosis	Survival without transplantation is usually until childhood only.	End stage disease usually between 50-70 years old. Good prognosis with dialysis.

Q: What are the clinical features of chronic renal failure?

Features may be considered as follows:

Features	Examples
Cardiovascular	Heart Failure, Hypertension, Pericarditis* & Peripheral Vascular Disease
Dermatological	Pale Yellow Skin & Pruritis*
Endocrine	Amenorrhoea, Impotence & Infertility
Fluid Overload	JVP Increase, Peripheral Oedema & Pulmonary Oedema
Gastrointestinal	Anorexia, Diarrhoea, Nausea & Vomiting*
Haematological	Anaemia, Ecchymosis & Epistaxis
Neurological	Confusion, Coma, Fits & Peripheral Neuropathy*
Respiratory	Halitosis & Pleural Effusion*
Surgical	Fistula & Nephrectomy Scar

* These features are commonly associated with uraemia.

Lower Gastrointestinal

Q: What is IBD?

Inflammatory bowel disease is an idiopathic inflammatory disease with a genetic predisposition & probable auto-immune component against the gastrointestinal tract. IBD is comprised of ulcerative colitis (UC) & Crohn's Disease (CD). Both are more prevalent in Ashkenazi Jews, followed by white Caucasian populations. Age of presentation peaks at around 20–30 years. Crohn's Disease is more prevalent in smokers, however ulcerative colitis is more prevalent in non-smokers.

Q: What are the intestinal presenting features of IBD?

Many features e.g. diarrhoea & mucus PR are similar, although UC features tend to be more severe than CD. Presenting features of CD may include growth retardation in children, anaemia, occult blood loss, low-grade fever & weight loss. UC often presents more acutely with abdominal pain, diarrhoea & frank blood loss PR. Severe acute exacerbations are also more prevalent in UC. Remember that CD features may be present throughout the entire gastrointestinal tract, whilst UC is limited to the colon.

Q: What features are characteristic of an acute exacerbation of UC?

- Abdominal Pain & Distension (may indicate perforated toxic megacolon)
- Bloody Stool
- Diarrhoea (>10 episodes in 24h)
- Faecal Urgency
- Pallor
- Pyrexia
- Tachycardia

Q: What investigations would assist in diagnosing IBD?

Investigation	Examples
Bloods	FBC, U&E & CRP
Radiology	AXR, Barium Enema & Small Bowel Follow Through
Procedures	Colonoscopy
Histology	Biopsy at Colonoscopy

Q: What differences may be seen between CD & UC on a barium enema?

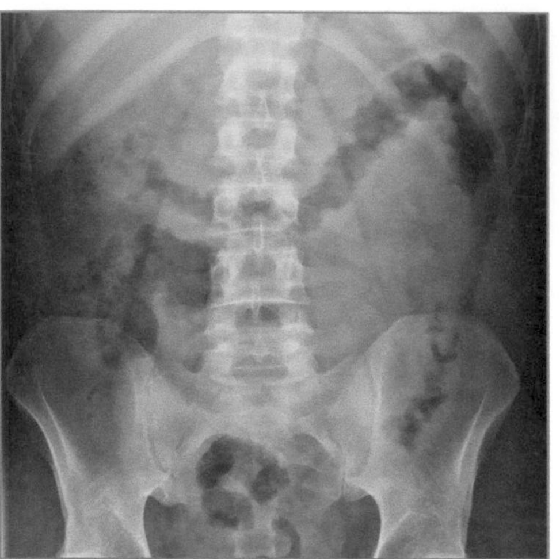

Fig 4.5: Ulcerative colitis radiography.

'Thumbprinting' is seen throughout the colon. This is due to thickening of the large bowel wall related to inflammation, with the normal haustra becoming thickened and prejecting into the aerated lumen.

Crohn's Disease	Ulcerative Colitis
String Sign (terminal ileum stricture)	Lead Piping (scarred, rigid colon)
Cobblestones / Skip Lesions	Loss of Haustration
Rose Thorn Ulcers	Toxic Megacolon

Q: What condition is shown in this barium enema & what is A, B & C?

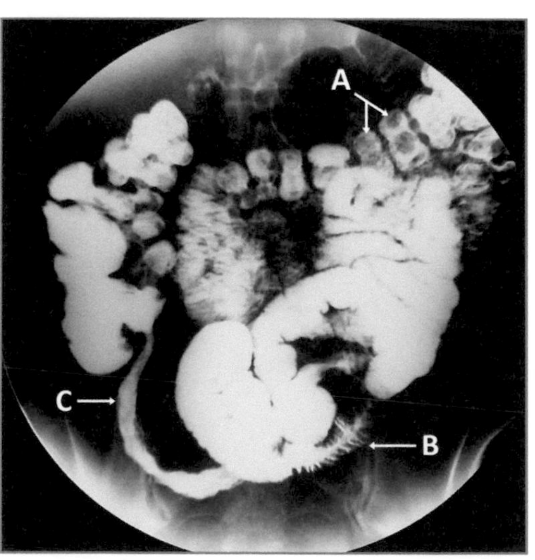

Fig 4.6: Barium enema of a patient with Crohn's Disease.

A: Cobblestones

B: Rose Thorn Ulcers

C: String Sign

Q: What are the pathological differences between CD & UC?

Features	Crohn's Disease	Ulcerative Colitis
MACROSCOPIC		
Pseudopolyps	√	√
Fistula	√	X
Stricture	√	X
Thick Wall	√	X
MICROSCOPIC		
Crypt Abscess	X	√
Granuloma	√	X
Inflammation	Patchy & Transmural	Continuous & Mucosal

Q: What are the complications of IBD?

These may be broadly classified according to IBD type as follows:

Crohn's Disease	Ulcerative Colitis
Infection	Infection
Failure to Thrive	Toxic Megacolon
Gastrointestinal Fistula	Primary Sclerosing Cholangitis*
Subacute Intestinal Obstruction	Colorectal Carcinoma

* PSC is present in 6–7% of patients with UC. UC is present in 60–70% of patients with PSC.

Q: What are the extra-intestinal associations of IBD?

- Mouth Ulcers (CD only)
- Perianal Skin Tags (CD only)
- Ankylosing Spondylitis
- Arthritis
- Iritis
- Erythema Nodosum
- Pyoderma Gangrenosum

Q: What are the treatment options for IBD?

Treatment	Crohn's Disease	Ulcerative Colitis
CONSERVATIVE	• Diet Modification • Psychological • Support Groups	• Psychological • Support Groups
MEDICAL	• Systemic Steroids • Immunosuppressants e.g. Azathioprine • Anti TNFα e.g. Infliximab	• Topical Steroids e.g. Predfoam Enemas • Systemic Steroids • 5-Aminosalicylic Acid e.g. Mesalazine
SURGICAL	• Drainage of Perianal Sepsis • Seton Fistulotomy • Stricturoplasty • Segmental Resection • Defunctioning Loop Ileostomy	• Proctocolectomy & End Ileostomy • Ileo-Anal Pouch Formation

Q: Is surgery for IBD curative?

UC may be cured by surgery, as the disease is limited to the colon. CD affects the entire gastrointestinal tract, so relapses may occur even after surgical intervention. Approximately 70% of CD patients & 30% of UC patients require surgery at some time.

Q: What are the indications for surgery in IBD?

Indication	Explanation	
Medical Treatment Complications	Patients who experience severe side effects from medical treatment.	
Medical Treatment Failure	Patients with IBD resistant to medical treatment.	
Disease Process Complications	**Acute:**	Abscess Fistula Toxic Megacolon
	Chronic:	Strictures Colonic Dysplasia (leading to carcinoma)

Q: What are the causes of an iliac fossa mass?

Skin & Soft Tissue	Gastrointestinal		Vascular
Cyst	***Right Iliac Fossa:***	***Left Iliac Fossa:***	Iliac Aneurysm
Lipoma	Caecal Carcinoma	Diverticulitis	Lymphadenopathy
Sarcoma	IBD	Faeces	
	Appendix		
Testicular	**Gynaecological**		**Urological**
Incomplete Descent	Benign Ovarian Tumour		Transplant Kidney
Ectopic Testis	Malignant Ovarian Tumour		
	Fibroids		

Rectum & Anus

Q: What is a sinus?

A blind ending tract extending from an epithelial defect. This may be normal e.g. cardiac, or pathological e.g. pilonidal sinus.

Q: What is a fistula & how can fistulae be classified?

An abnormal communication between 2 epithelial surfaces. The most common fistula is traumatically acquired as an ear piercing! Fistulae may be classified as follows:

Iatrogenic	Congenital	Acquired
Trauma e.g. Bowel Resection	Parkes-Weber Syndrome	Trauma e.g. Ear Piercing
Cimino-Brescia Fistula	Tracheo-Oesophageal	Infective e.g. TB / Perianal
		Inflammatory e.g. CD
		Neoplastic

Q: What is the cryptoglandular sepsis theory?

An anorectal abscess is a discrete soft tissue infection around the anus. The severity & depth is highly variable. The cavity of the abscess may discharge in a manner associated with formation of a fistulous tract. The cryptoglandular sepsis theory attributes a particular level of anal fistula development from a particular level of anorectal abscess as follows:

Anorectal Abscess	Corresponding Anal Fistula
Perianal	**Subcutaneous / Submucous**
Intersphincteric	**Intersphincteric**
Ischiorectal	**High Anal** (involves both anal sphincters)
	Low Anal (involves internal anal sphincter only)
Supralevator	**Pelvirectal** (above anorectal ring)

Q: How would you manage a patient with a perianal abscess?

- **Full History:** Is there as history of IBD, previous abscesses or immunosuppression e.g. diabetes, steroids, immunosuppressants or HIV?
- **Thorough Clinical Examination** including PR examination.
- **Proctoscopy / Sigmoidoscopy:** To seek internal fistula opening if present.
- **Surgery:** GA incision & drainage, sending pus for MC&S. Once deroofed, irrigate, deloculate, wash & pack the abscess to assist healing by secondary intention. Do not explore for a fistula acutely.
- **Clinic Follow-up:** If MC&S confirms presence of intestinal bacteria, suspect a fistula & arrange further investigation e.g. MRI, or treatment as necessary.

Q: You order an MRI of a patient with gastrointestinal flora at MC&S from a sample of pus taken at incision & drainage of an anal abscess. This demonstrates an anal fistula. What surgical treatment options are available?

These depend on the level & severity of the fistula as follows:

Procedure	Fistula
Lay Open	Subcutaneous, Submucous & Low Anal
Seton	High Anal & Intersphincteric
Fistulotomy & Flap	Complicated Fistulae

Q: What is Goodsall's Rule?

This describes the predictable course of an anal fistula, governed by its external opening (Fig 4.7). The patient is put in the lithotomy position & a line is imagined through 3 & 9 o'clock. Fistulae with external openings above this line form a radial tract directly to the same position internally. Fistulae with external openings below this line open in the posterior midline by horseshoeing through an unpredictable course.

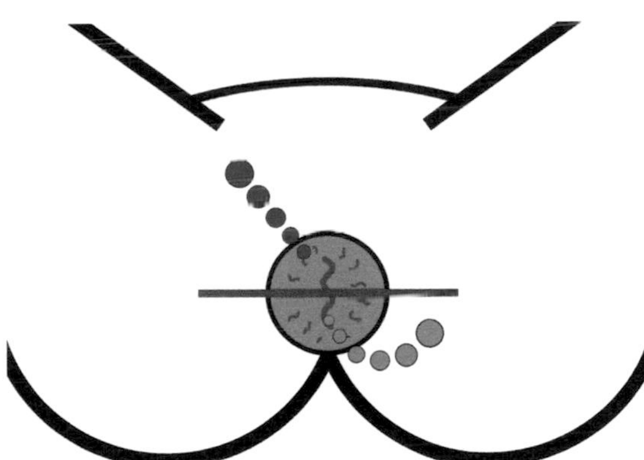

Fig 4.7: Goodsall's Rule.

Imagine line through 3 & 9 o'clock in lithotomy position.

External opening above line = direct course to internal opening.

External opening below line = horseshoeing course to midline internal opening.

Common Abdominal Scars

Q: Can you draw some common abdominal scars?

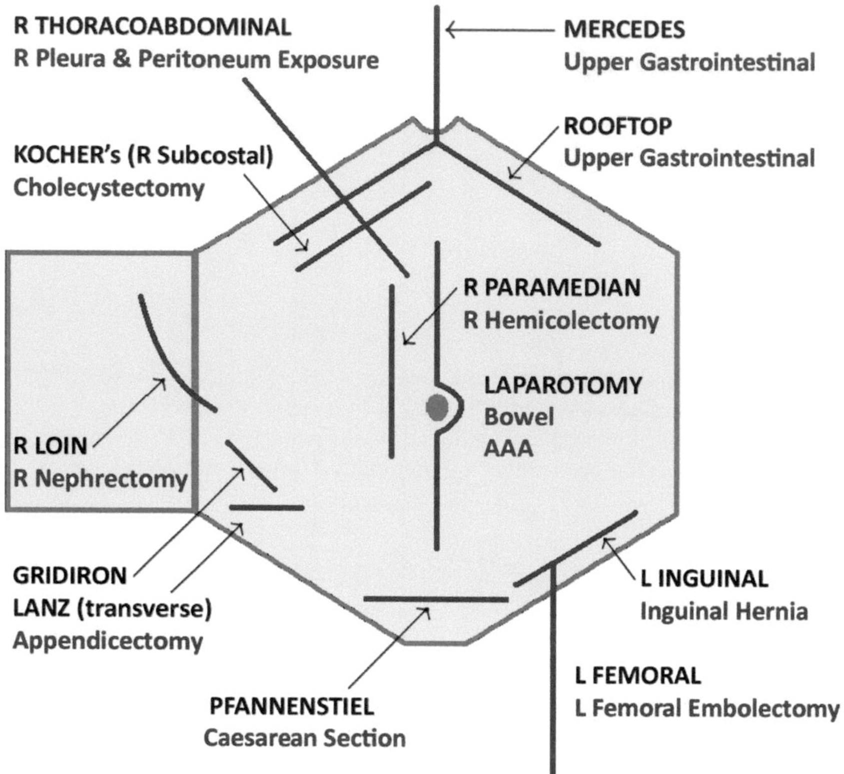

Fig 4.8: Diagram of common abdominal scars. Note the right thoracoabdominal, midline laparotomy & left femoral incisions are labelled but not arrowed. **Red labelling indicates the potential reason for making the incision.**

CHAPTER 5
HERNIAE & SCROTUM

BH Miranda
MJ Portou
MC Winslet

CHAPTER CONTENTS

Hernia Examination

Scrotal Lump Examination

OSCE Questions

- Herniae
- Testicular Maldescent
- Benign Scrotal Lumps
- Testicular Torsion
- Testicular Tumours

HERNIA EXAMINATION

START: The patient should be standing, fully exposed from umbilicus to knees.

Chaperone is vital.

Examine the groin lump / hernia, kneeling at the side of the patient.

Inspection	Interpretation
6 x S's	Describe lump site, size, shape, symmetry, overlying skin & associated scars.
Cough Impulse	Ask the patient to cough & check for an impulse.

Ask about pain.

Check for temperature changes, using the back of your hand.

Ask the patient if the lump is reducible.

If reduction of the hernia is not possible with the patient standing, assist them with lying down so they may reduce the hernia, then continue the examination with the patient standing again.

Palpation may be divided into 4 steps:

Palpation	Interpretation
Step 1 ***'SEC FFP TR'***	Palpate lump surface, edge, consistency, fixity to skin & underlying structures, fluctuance, pulsatility & expansility, transilluminability & reducibility.
Step 2	Delineate anatomy (Fig 5.1). • Inguinal herniae emerge above & medial to the pubic tubercle. • Femoral herniae emerge below & lateral to the pubic tubercle.
Step 3	Ask the patient to reduce the lump & place the palmar surfaces of 2 fingertips over the superficial ring. Ask the patient to cough, then note if an 'impulse' is felt. Next remove your fingertips & ask the patient to cough again. • Indirect inguinal herniae will be contained at the superficial ring. • Direct inguinal herniae will reappear lateral to the controlled superficial ring.
Step 4	Ask the patient to reduce the lump & assist the patient in 'milking' the inguinal canal from the superficial to deep ring. Place the palmar surfaces of 2 fingertips over the deep ring & ask the patient to cough. Note if an 'impulse' is felt. Now remove your fingertips & ask the patient to cough again. • Indirect inguinal herniae will be controlled at the deep ring. • Direct inguinal herniae will reappear medial to the controlled deep ring.

Ausculation	Interpretation
Bowel Sounds	Herniae may contain bowel. This includes indirect inguinoscrotal herniae so do not forget to auscultate a scrotal lump!

Completion	Interpretation
Lymphadenopathy	Palpate for inguinal lymphadenopathy.
Contralateral Side	There may be an associated lesion.
Scrotum	There may be an associated lesion.
Abdominal Exam	Full abdominal examination is important, particularly in the acute stage, where incarceration & strangulation may precipitate abdominal pain & change in bowel habit.

FINISH:

SCROTAL LUMP EXAMINATION

START: The patient should be standing, fully exposed from umbilicus to knees.

Chaperone is vital.

Examine the scrotal lump, kneeling at the side of the patient.

Inspection	Interpretation
6 x S's	Describe lump site, size, shape, symmetry, overlying skin & associated scars.
Cough Impulse	Ask the patient to cough & check for an impulse. This may indicate an indirect inguinal-scrotal hernia rather than a true scrotal lesion.

Ask about pain.

Check for temperature changes, using the back of your hand.

Ask the patient if the lump is reducible.

Palpation	Interpretation
SEC FFP TR	Palpate lump surface, edge, consistency, fixity to skin & underlying structures, fluctuance, pulsatility & expansility, transilluminability & reducibility.
Get Above The Lump?	This is a vital step in the examination. If one can't get above a scrotal lump, it is likely to be an indirect inguinal-scrotal hernia. If one can get above the lump, it is likely to be a true scrotal lump.
Testicle	The testicle should be palpated as a separate structure.
Epididymis	The epididymis should be palpated as a separate structure.
Vas Deferens	The vas deferens should be palpated as a separate structure.

If you can't get above the lump, continue palpation as for a groin / hernia lump from STEP 2.

If you can get above the lump, continue the scrotal lump examination as outlined below.

Completion	Interpretation
Lymphadenopathy	Palpate for lymphadenopathy. Remember that the penis & skin of the scrotum drain to inguinal nodes. Remember that the testes drain to retroperitoneal para-aortic nodes that may be enlarged but not palpable.
Contralateral Side	There may be an associated lesion.

FINISH:

OSCE QUESTIONS

Herniae

Q: Can you delineate the hernia relevant anatomy of the inguinal region?

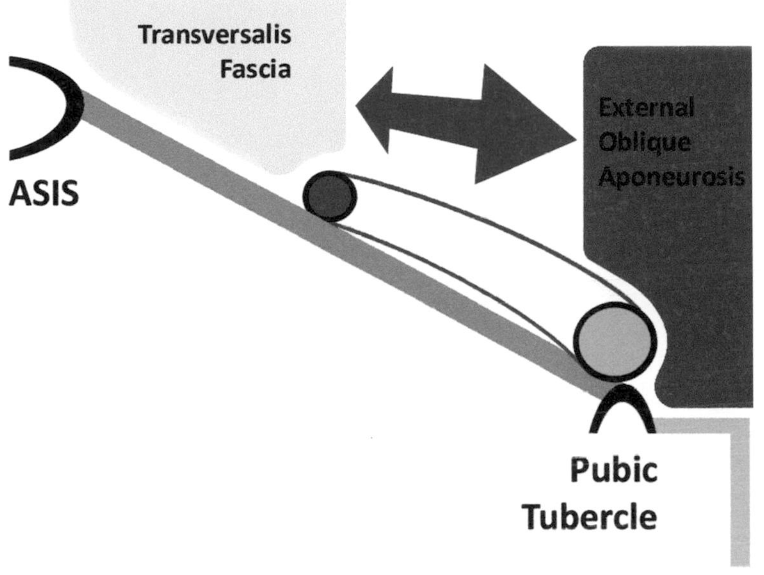

Fig 5.1: Hernia relevant anatomy of the right inguinal region *(see colour coding below).*

Anatomy	Notes
ASIS & Pubic Tubercle	The anterior superior iliac spine (ASIS) & pubic tubercles must be identified first.
Inguinal Ligament	Delineate the inguinal ligament which has attachments to both the anterior superior iliac spine (ASIS) & pubic tubercle.
Deep Ring	Point out the location of the deep ring which lies just above the midpoint of the inguinal ligament. It is formed by an aperture through the transversalis fascia. Mention that the femoral artery may be palpated below the inguinal ligament at the mid-inguinal point, halfway between the ASIS & pubic symphysis.
Superficial Ring	Point out the location of the superficial ring which lies just above the pubic tubercle. It is formed by an aperture through the **external oblique aponeurosis**.
Inguinal Canal	Finally, explain that the inguinal canal is an oblique communication between the deep & superficial inguinal rings, formed by the arching fibres of the **transversus abdominis** & **internal oblique** muscles.

Q: What are the borders of the inguinal canal?

Border	Anatomy
Posterior Wall	Transversalis Fascia
Anterior Wall	External Oblique Aponeurosis
Floor	Inguinal Ligament
Roof	Arching Fibres of Transversus Abdominis & Internal Oblique

Q: What are the differential diagnoses of a groin lump?

These include the differential diagnoses of any lump *(see lumps 'n' bumps chapter)* and those specific to the groin as follows:

Above the Inguinal Ligament	Below the Inguinal Ligament
Inguinal Hernia	Femoral Hernia
Testicular Maldescent	Testicular Maldescent
	Saphena Varix
	Femoral Artery Aneurysm

Q: What are the differential diagnoses of a scrotal lump?

These include the differential diagnoses of any lump *(see lumps 'n' bumps chapter)* & those specific to the contents of the scrotum. With respect to scrotal contents, differential diagnoses may be classified according to findings on palpation as follows:

Can't Get Above Lump	
Indirect Inguinal-Scrotal Hernia	
Congenital / Infantile Hydrocoele	
Can Get Above Lump & Palpable Separately to Testis	**Can Get Above Lump & Palpable With the Testis**
Epididymal Cyst	Haematocoele
Epididymitis	Hydrocoele
Spermatocoele	Orchitis
Varicocoele	Torsion
	Tumour

Q: What is an inguinal hernia?

An abnormal protrusion of abdominal contents through the inguinal region (Fig 5.2). It is the most common groin hernia & may be classified as direct / indirect as follows:

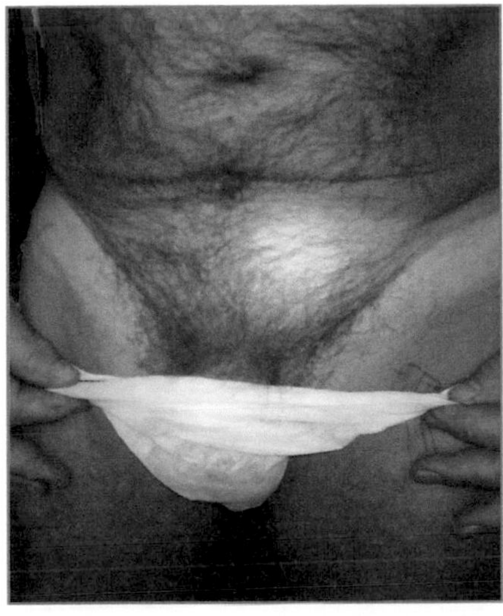

Fig 5.2: Left-sided indirect inguinal hernia.

Classification	Notes
Direct	Due to an acquired weakness in the transversalis fascia. Increased incidence with age, COPD, obesity & smoking. The hernia protrudes directly through the weakness (Hesselbach's Triangle), without traversing the inguinal canal.
Indirect	Due to a patent processus vaginalis. This is a congenital defect which allows for the hernia to traverse the deep ring, inguinal canal & superficial ring. If extension into the scrotum is observed, an indirect inguinoscrotal hernia is present.

Q: What are the treatment options for an inguinal hernia?

Treatment	Examples
Conservative	A truss is a device that may be used to help contain an easily reducible inguinal hernia within the abdomen, however it is not curative & rarely required.
Medical	Optimise COPD medication & treat pneumonia to prevent coughing which increases intra-abdominal pressure & may worsen the hernia.
Surgical	This is the gold standard treatment. It involves surgical herniotomy & herniorrhaphy that may be performed laparoscopically or open. **Lichtenstein's Repair** involves the use of a polypropylene mesh to reinforce the repair. If there is any concern about associated infection, **Shouldice's Repair** may be preferred as this does not involve the use of a mesh. Instead, a 4 layer overlapping muscle repair is undertaken.

Q: What is a femoral hernia?

An abnormal protrusion through the femoral canal. It is less common than an inguinal hernia. It is seen more commonly in females due to stretching of the femoral canal during pregnancy, or fat regression within the femoral canal after menopause.

Q: What are the treatment options for a femoral hernia?

There is no place for conservative management of a femoral hernia due to the high risk of incarceration & strangulation. All femoral herniae should therefore be operated on as soon as possible. Asymptomatic, reducible femoral herniae may be operated on using a low approach e.g. **Lockwood's Repair**. Symptomatic, strangulated femoral herniae may be operated on using a high approach e.g. **McEvedy's Repair**, which may easily be extended to a laparotomy to resect dead bowel if necessary.

Q: Do you know of any other herniae?

Hernia	Notes
Littre's	Containing a Meckel's Diverticulum.
Maydl's	Containing a 'W' shaped loop of bowel, such that the middle arm of the 'W' becomes compressed & strangulated.
Richter's	Containing only one side of the bowel wall, which may become strangulated.
Sliding	Part of the hernia sac wall is composed of bowel. This is also known as a hernia *'en glissade'*.
Epigastric	Abnormal protrusion of abdominal contents through the epigastric region of the linea alba. Surgery includes herniotomy & herniorrhaphy, with repair of the defective linea alba either directly or with a reinforcing mesh.
Incisional	Abnormal protrusion of abdominal contents through a weakness in the abdominal wall, at a site of previous surgery. The underlying aetiology is therefore iatrogenic. It is rarely symptomatic & risk of strangulation is low, so conservative treatment is often all that is required. Surgical options include tension free mesh repair either laparoscopically or open.
Spigelian	Abnormal protrusion of abdominal contents through the linea semilunaris. Open or laparoscopic mesh repair is advocated due to the risk of strangulation.

Hernia	Notes
Umbilical	Abnormal protrusion of abdominal contents through a defect of / near the cicatrix. It may be congenital or acquired (Fig 5.3). If congenital, it is due to a congenital defect of closure & includes the following: 1. **Exomphalos:** Herniation of abdominal contents, covered by a transparent membrane composed of 3 layers. The outer layer is amniotic membrane, the middle layer Wharton's Jelly & the inner layer peritoneum. There is a risk of perforation & peritonitis, so surgical repair is required. 2. **Gastroschisis:** Herniation of abdominal contents just lateral to the cicatrix, without a covering membrane. Hypothermia, hypovolaemia & sepsis may occur due to the presence of eviscerated bowel. Immediate treatment involves placement of a NGT, fluid resuscitation & protection of bowel with sterile packs & bags. Surgical repair is then required.
Paraumbilical	Abnormal protrusion of abdominal contents through a defect in the *linea alba* near the umbilicus. There is a high risk of strangulation. Surgical options include a Mayo repair, or repair of the defect using a reinforcing mesh. A Mayo repair involves herniotomy & herniorrhaphy, repairing the defect by suturing the upper part of rectus over the lower part of rectus in a *'vest over pants'* fashion.
Brainstem	Due to increased intracranial pressure e.g. post head injury.
Diaphragmatic	Hiatus hernia. (Fig 5.4)

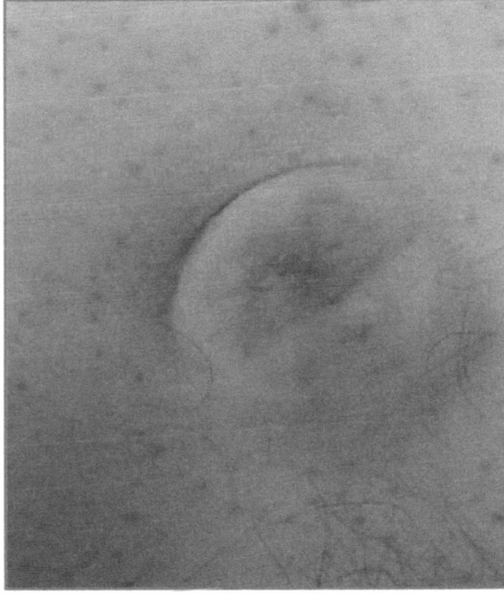

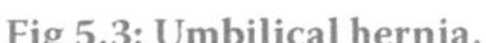

Fig 5.3: Umbilical hernia.

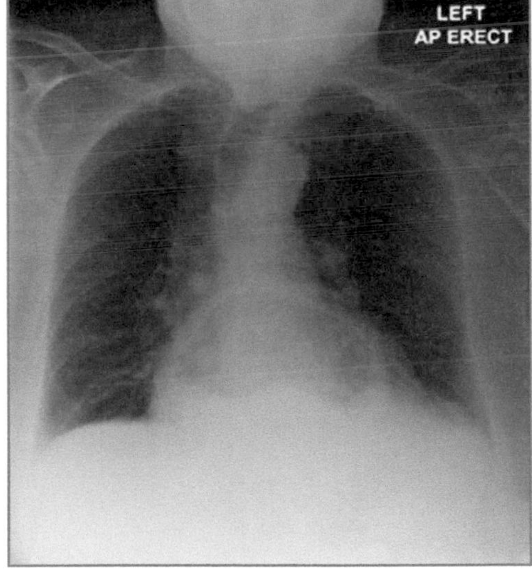

Fig 5.4: Hiatus hernia radiograph

A supra-diaphragmatic 'mass' is visible with an air-fluid level. This represents a hiatus hernia. There is also a left humerus fracture noted.

Testicular Maldescent

Q: What is testicular maldescent?

This terminology encompasses 3 abnormalities of descent of the testis as follows:

Abnormality	Notes
Retractile	This is due to an overactive cremasteric reflex & affects children. The testis appears to be incompletely descended, but may be noticed within the scrotum after a warm bath. Treatment is conservative as the testis becomes less retractile with age.
Ectopic	The testis descends to an abnormal position after exiting the superficial inguinal ring. Common locations include the superficial inguinal pouch, perineum, root of penis & within the femoral canal.
Undescended Testis	The undescended testis prematurely stops its descent anywhere along the normal path of descent as guided by the gubernaculum.

Q: What are the complications of an undescended testis?

Complications include an increased risk of:

- Trauma
- Torsion
- Tumour
- Infertility
- Psychological Distress

Undescended testes confer a 30X risk of developing a testicular tumour, most commonly a seminoma. Treatment consists of early orchidopexy.

Q: What is the treatment for an undescended testis?

Orchidopexy is the treatment of choice & this should be undertaken at the age of 1 year to prevent complications. If an undescended testis is noticed in an older child, a short course of hCG or GnRH may help in approximately 15% of cases.

Benign Scrotal Lumps

Q: What is a hydrocoele?

This is a scrotal swelling due to fluid accumulation within the tunica vaginalis & may be classified as follows:

Classification	Explanation
Primary	Due to a persistent processus vaginalis.
Secondary	Occurs in response to underlying disease e.g. infection, torsion & tumour.

Q: What types of primary hydrocoeles do you know of?

Primary Hydrocoele	Notes
Vaginal	This is the most common primary hydrocoele. Accumulation of fluid is limited to the tunica vaginalis & neither extends to the vas deferens, nor communicates with the peritoneal cavity.
Congenital	Accumulation of fluid extends to surround the vas deferens. There is also communication with the peritoneal cavity as the processus vaginalis is not obliterated.
Infantile	Accumulation of fluid extends to surround the vas deferens. The processus vaginalis is obliterated at the level of the deep ring, so there is no communication with the peritoneal cavity.
Hydrocoele of the Cord	This is rare. Accumulation of fluid is limited to vas deferens only.

Q: What treatment options are available for a hydrocoele?

Infants with a hydrocoele may be managed conservatively until the age of 1 year when surgery is indicated. Secondary hydrocoeles resolve with treatment of the underlying cause. Treatment options for primary hydrocoeles may therefore be classified as follows:

Conservative	Surgical
Reassurance	**Aspirate:** This is both therapeutic & diagnostic.
Scrotal Support	**Phenol Injection:** Phenol is a sclerosing agent that may prevent recurrence.
	Lord's Plication: The hydrocoele sac is incised & plicated behind the testis.
	Jaboulay's Procedure: The hydrocoele sac is incised, partially excised & the remaining tissue is plicated behind the testis.

Q: What are epididymitis & orchitis?

Epididymitis is inflammation of the epididymis. Orchitis is inflammation of the testicle. Clinical features include acute pain, erythema & oedema. Clinical features of a urinary tract & systemic infection may also be present. Acute cases may progress to chronic, especially when TB is the cause.

Q: What are the causes of epididymitis & orchitis?

Cause	Examples
Viral	Mumps, Infectious Mononucleosis & Coxsackie B
Bacterial	Ascending UTI e.g. *E. coli*, STD e.g. *Chlamydia*, TB

Q: What is important about an acute presentation of epididymitis & orchitis?

It is important to differentiate this from torsion. Thorough history & clinical examination should point towards an infective cause rather than torsion. **If in any doubt, explore the scrotum**. The following investigations assist in diagnosis:

Investigation	Examples
Haematology & Biochemistry	FBC, U&E & CRP.
Serology	VDRL.
Microbiology	• **Swabs** for MC+S. • **MSU** for MC+S. • **3 x Early Morning Urine Samples for ZN Staining & Microscopy:** The presence of acid-fast bacilli indicates TB.
Radiology	USS.

Q: What are the treatment options for epididymitis & orchitis?

Treatment	Acute	Chronic
CONSERVATIVE	Bed Rest & Scrotal Support	Bed Rest & Scrotal Support
MEDICAL	Analgesia	Analgesia
	Antibiotics e.g. Ciprofloxacin	Antibiotics e.g. anti-TB regimen
SURGICAL	Abscess Drainage	Orchidectomy if severe

Q: What are epididymal cysts?

Fluid filled swellings of the epididymis which are palpated separately from the testes. They are often multiple, fluctuant & transilluminate. Large persistent cysts may be excised.

Q: What is a spermatocoele?

A cystic swelling that contains spermatozoa. It is most commonly found at the epididymis & spermatic cord. Clinical features & treatment are similar to epididymal cysts.

Q: What is a varicocoele?

A collection of dilated tortuous veins of the pampiniform plexus. Clinically, the scrotum appears as a 'bag of worms' when the patient is standing. This appearance disappears when the patient is lying. 98% are left sided as the left testicular vein (longer than the right) drains directly into the left renal vein (may be compressed where it is crossed by the colon). Varicocoeles appearing in late adulthood should be investigated further for possible invasion of the left renal vein by carcinoma. If symptomatic, surgical treatment options include radiological embolisation & ligation of the testicular vein proximal to the deep inguinal ring, either open or laparoscopically.

Testicular Torsion

Q: What is testicular torsion & why does it occur?

This is an acute condition where the testicle twists around the axis of the spermatic cord. It often affects teenagers & young adults, with a recent history of trauma, who may have an underlying abnormality. The **bell clapper** testicular abnormality describes a tunica vaginalis that doesn't anchor to the testicle, hence allowing free movement of the testicle like the clapper inside a bell.

Q: What are the clinical features of testicular torsion & how would you manage it?

Clinical features include an acutely hot, painful & tender scrotal swelling, abdominal pain, nausea & vomiting. The cord may be shorter & thicker than the contralateral side on palpation, due to twisting along its axis. This is a surgical emergency & there is only a 4–6 hour window in which to salvage the testicle. Management strategies include:

- Appropriate Resuscitation
- NBM
- FBC, U&E, G&S
- (IV) Fluids
- Analgesia
- Consent Patient for Scrotal Exploration +/- Bilateral Orchidopexy +/- Orchidectomy
- Place Patient on Emergency List
- Inform Anaesthetist

Q: What are the differential diagnoses for testicular torsion?

- Epididymitis & Orchitis
- Hydatid of Morgagni Torsion
- Strangulated Inguinal Hernia

Testicular Tumours

Q: What testicular tumours do you know of?

Classification	Examples	Notes
BENIGN	**Leydig Cell Tumour**	Benign neoplasm of interstitial Leydig cells. May cause precocious puberty due to secretion of testosterone.
	Sertoli Cell Tumour	Benign neoplasm of Sertoli cells. May cause gynaecomastia due to release of oestrogens.
MALIGNANT	**Seminoma**	Malignant neoplasm of seminiferous tubule cells with a peak age of 30-40 years. Represents approximately 40% of testicular malignancy. Teratomas may secrete βhCG (never αFP).
	Teratoma	Malignant neoplasm containing elements from all 3 germ layers, derived from multipotent cells that display a wide range of differentiation. Represents approximately 30% of testicular malignancy. Teratomas may secrete αFP & βhCG.
	Mixed	Malignant neoplasm composed of both seminoma & teratoma. Represents approximately 20% of testicular malignancy.
	Lymphoma **Choriocarcinoma** **Gonadoblastoma**	Together represent approximately 10% of testicular malignancies.

Q: What are the clinical features of testicular malignancy?

- Painless, Hard Testicular Lump
- Sensation of Dragging
- Secondary Hydrocoele
- Back Pain (para-aortic lymphadenopathy)
- Respiratory Features (lung metastases)

Q: What staging systems do you know of for testicular malignancy?

Royal Marsden Staging:

Stage	Definition
I	Tumour confined to testis.
II	Para-aortic lymphadenopathy.
III	Supra-diaphragmatic lymphadenopathy.
IV	Extra-nodal matastases.
L	**L1:** <3 lung metastases. **L2:** >3 lung metastases all <2cm in diameter. **L3:** >3 lung metastases with ≥1 lesions >2cm in diameter.
H	Liver metastases.

TNM Classification:

Tumour Spread (T)	
Tx:	Tumour can't be assessed.
T0:	No tumour present.
Tis:	Carcinoma *in situ*.
T1:	Tumour confined to testicle or epididymis.
T2:	Tumour confined to testicle or epididymis but either with local Invasion of the tunica albuginea, vessels or lymph nodes.
T3:	Tumour invades the spermatic cord.
T4:	Tumour invades the scrotum.

Regional Lymphadenopathy (N)	
N0:	No regional lymphadenopathy.
N1:	Regional lymphadenopathy <2cm in diameter.
N2:	Regional lymphadenopathy 2-5 cm in diameter.
N3:	Regional lymphadenopathy >5cm in diameter.

Distant Metastasis or Lymphadenopathy (M)	
M0:	No regional lymphadenopathy.
M1a:	Lung metastases or distant lymphadenopathy.
M1b:	Any other organ metastases.

Q: What investigations would you consider for a patient with a suspected testicular malignancy?

Investigations	Notes
Blood Tests	αFP, βhCG & LDH
Radiology	• **Scrotal USS:** Tumour assessment • **CXR:** Lung metastases • **CT:** Staging of disease

Q: What happens to αFP & βhCG levels in testicular tumours?

Tumour	Biochemistry
Seminoma	Raised βhCG
Non Seminoma • Teratoma • Yolk Sac Tumours	Raised αFP Raised βhCG

Q: What treatment options are there for testicular malignancy?

Treatment depends on underlying pathology & includes:

Treatment	Notes
Surgery	Orchidectomy via an inguinal approach, after clamping the cord. A scrotal incision is avoided to prevent seeding to scrotal skin that is drained by inguinal lymph nodes (not para-aortic).
Chemotherapy	Seminoma & Teratoma.
Radiotherapy	Seminoma.

CHAPTER 6
STOMA

BH Miranda
MJ Portou
MC Winslet

CHAPTER CONTENTS

Stoma Examination

OSCE Questions

STOMA EXAMINATION

START: Patient exposure is to underwear ideally. This also allows for further examination of the abdominal system.

The stoma may initially be examined with the patient standing, followed by lying flat.

The stoma bag should be taken off to allow for a thorough examination of the operation site & bag constituents.

Use sheet covers appropriately, to maintain patient dignity.

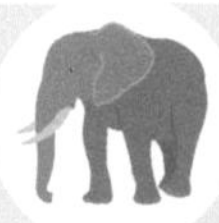

Memory: 'Small Bags Should Lay More Snugly On Committed Patients'

INSPECTION	Interpretation
Site	Ideally should be sited away from bony prominences, scars & skin folds. Common stoma sites include: • **Epigastric** = PEG & Transverse Loop Colostomy. • **Right Iliac Fossa** = Iliostomy (Fig 6.1). • **Left Iliac Fossa** = Colostomy.
Bag & Contents	• **Fluid** = Small Bowel Contents (Iliostomy) / Urine (Urostomy). • **Solid** = Large Bowel Contents (Colostomy).
Spout?	• **Spout Present** = Iliostomy (Fig 6.1). • **Flush to Skin** = Colostomy.
Lumen	• **1 Lumen** = End Iliostomy (Fig 6.1). • **2 Lumens** = Loop Iliostomy.
Mucosa	Comment on whether the mucosa is healthy or unhealthy e.g. inflamed or ulcerated.
Scar	Comment on associated scars that may indicate the underlying procedure.
Old Sites	Comment on scars that may indicate previous stoma formation e.g. Crohn's Disease.
Complications	Comment on presence of complications as follows: • **Anatomical** = Prolapse, Retraction, Stenosis & Parastomal Hernia (ask the patient to cough). • **Dermatological** = Skin Discomfort & Excoriations Present (primarily due to leakage of iliostomy contents). • **Metabolic** = Electrolyte Imbalance. • **Vascular** = Haemorrhage, Ischaemia & Gangrene. • **Psychological** = Psychosexual Disturbance. • **Other** = Associated Gallstone Disease.
Perineum	The anus will be absent in an AP resection.

Ask about pain.

Look at the patient's face throughout the examination.

Warm your hands by rubbing them together & warn the patient that they may be cold.

Feel for any temperature changes with the back of your hand.

PALPATION	Interpretation
Lumen	Place a finger into the lumen to ensure adequate patency.
Parastomal Hernia	This must be specifically palpated & may have a cough impulse.
Stoma Bag	Comment on the stoma bag as follows: • **1 x Piece** = The whole bag must be changed as 1 unit. • **2 x Piece** = There is a base plate on the skin & only the bag must be changed.

AUSCULTATION	Interpretation
Bowel Sounds	• Comment on presence or absence of bowel sounds e.g. Ileus (absent). • Comment on character of bowel sounds e.g. Bowel Obstruction (tinkling).

COMPLETION	Interpretation
Abdominal Examination	A full abdominal examination is vital *(see abdomen chapter)*.

FINISH:

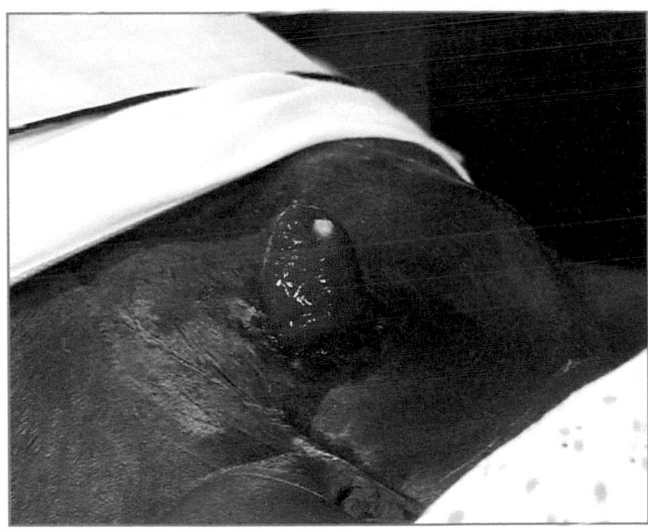

Fig 6.1: Active end ileostomy. Note the laparotomy scar & transverse scar from previous stoma formation.

OSCE QUESTIONS

Q: What is an enteric surgical stoma?

This is an iatrogenic opening that connects part of the bowel to the outside world. In the case of enteric stomas, a bag is required to collect the resulting discharge.

Q: How would you classify enteric surgical stomas?

These may be classified as end / loop & ileostomy / colostomy as follows:

Classification	Ileostomy	Colostomy
End	Panproctocolectomy	Hartmann's Procedure (rectosigmoid emergencies) AP Resection
Loop	Diversion Protect Distal Anastomosis	Palliative Diversion (pre-chemo / radiotherapy)

Q: What are the clinical indications for an enteric surgical stoma?

Indications	Notes
Feeding	Enteral feeding is preferred to TPN e.g. PEG & PEJ.
Diversion	Temporarily protects distal bowel with view to later reversal e.g. defunctioning loop ileostomy. In these cases, primary bowel anastomosis may be contraindicated or a distal abscess / fistula may be present.
Lavage	Temporary stomas for on-table lavage prior to bowel resection.
Operation	Hartmann's Procedure fashions a temporary colostomy that may be later reversed e.g. rectosigmoid emergencies. Other examples include AP Resection & Panproctocolectomy, when permanent stomas are required.

SECTION A3: LIMBS, SPINE & VASCULAR

CHAPTER 7
ORTHOPAEDICS

S Kamalasekaran
AD Ebinesan
BH Miranda
J Saksena

CHAPTER CONTENTS

Musculoskeletal Examination Tips

Orthopaedic Neck Examination

Spine Examination

Shoulder Examination

Elbow Examination

Hip Examination

Knee Examination

Ankle / Foot Examination

OSCE Questions

- Gait
- Osteoarthritis
- Rheumatoid Arthritis
- Ankylosing Spondylitis
- Paget's Disease of Bone
- Painful Shoulder
- Ankle & Foot Pathology

MUSCULOSKELETAL EXAMINATION TIPS

Scars, Swellings, Symmetry, Deformity, Erythema, Sinus, Muscle Wasting

As with all examination protocols, the key to success is to look slick & efficient! It is useful to have a standard introduction strategy when you 'look' at the patient. The above 7 clinical signs should be rehearsed in succession by the candidate, until they literally 'trips off the tongue'.

When examining a joint from all sides, the candidate will therefore be able to examine (e.g. the front, back & sides of the joint) for all of these signs in 1 movement around the patient. Examining for each of these 7 signs from the front, then each of these 7 signs from the sides, then each of these 7 signs from the back, takes longer & looks less slick!

This is particularly noticeable when the candidate is asked to comment as they go through the examination process. Rather than repeating each of the 7 signs (e.g. from the front, then sides, then back), the candidate can move around the patient with 1 movement, using a line as follows:

"I am examining the joint from the front, back & sides, for any scars, swellings, symmetry, deformity, erythema, sinuses & muscle wasting."

As with all examinations, if an obvious lump is seen, it should be inspected according to the *6 x S's (see lumps 'n' bumps chapter)*, prior to looking at the rest of the joint. Furthermore it should be palpated, prior to feeling the rest of the joint.

Like-for-Like

When testing power in any clinical examination, it is important (as far as possible) to test like-for-like, such that the same limbs & muscles are being used by the patient & examiner. This is to ensure that as much bias is removed as possible, due to discrepancies in patient–examiner muscle strength. For example, when testing elbow flexion of the right arm, the examiner should use flexion of their right elbow also.

Compare Each Side

Comparing each side assists in diagnosis of pathology that is either unilateral / worse on 1 side. This is always important. Furthermore, as it is not always possible to compare like-for-like, sometimes the only indication of pathology may be an imbalance between clinical signs on both sides e.g. left vs. right leg.

Valgus vs. Varus Deformity

Remember that these joint deformities are defined by the relationship of the distal joint.

- Valgus deformity implies that the distal joint is deviated away from the midline.
- Varus deformity implies that the distal joint is deviated towards the midline.

ORTHOPAEDIC NECK EXAMINATION

START: Patient sitting on chair, shirt off / exposed to level below the clavicles.

Inspect from FRONT, BACK & SIDES as follows:

LOOK	Interpretation
Scars	Post-operative, post-infective.
Swelling	Soft tissue / bony mass. Remember to check the thyroid region separately. Also look in the supraclavicular fossae for fullness e.g. Pancoast tumour.
Symmetry	Torticollis (involuntary neck contractions result in head tilting towards the side of the precipitating lesion / underlying pathology).
Deformity	Kyphosis / loss of normal lordosis. Vertebral collapse due to e.g. fracture, TB or tumour. Klippel-Feil Syndrome (patients have a low hairline, shortened webbed neck & decreased cervical spine ROM due to variable vertebral fusion).
Erythema	Inflammation.
Sinus	Post-operative, Infective.
Muscle Wasting	Previous trauma, neurological or infection e.g. TB.

Ask about pain.

To prevent causing distress, explain to the patient that you will be standing behind them.

Remember to feel the vertebrae, sides & front of the neck including the supraclavicular fossae.

Feel for temperature changes with the back of your hand.

FEEL	Interpretation
Tenderness	Feel midline structures, then paraspinal muscles, from occiput to C7/T1. **Note: The most prominent spinous process is that of T1 not C7 (vertebra prominens).** Tenderness in an isolated intervertebral space may be associated with cervical spondylosis.
Stepping	Run fingers down the midline of the spine from occiput to C7/T1. Feel for an abnormal 'step' that may be due to previous trauma, tumour or infection.
Mass	Soft tissue / bony mass. Remember to check the thyroid region separately.
Cervical Rib	Feel in the supraclavicular fossae for a cervical rib.
Lymph Nodes	Infection e.g. TB *(see head & neck chapter).*

Listen / feel for crepitations during movement.

Repeat movements with downward pressure on head. Intervertebral foramen stenosis may be amplified, hence reproducing associated neurological symptoms.

MOVE	Interpretation
Flexion	Ask patient to touch chin to chest & record chin–chest distance. Normal = 80°.
Extension	Ask patient to look up at the ceiling. The plane of the nose & forehead should be horizontal. Normal = 50°.
Lateral Flexion	Ask patient to touch ear to shoulder on both sides. ROM commonly decreased in cervical spondylosis. Normal = 45°.
Rotation	Ask patient to look over shoulder on both sides, whilst standing behind patient & stabilising the contralateral shoulder. Normal = 80°.

SPECIAL TEST	Interpretation
Thoracic Outlet Syndrome *(also see thoracic outlet syndrome in vascular chapter)*	1. **Hand Ischemia:** Look for signs e.g. cold, discolouration & trophic changes. 2. **Roo's Test (Fig 7.1):** With the patient sitting in a chair, position the patient's arms in 90° shoulder abduction & full external rotation, with the elbow flexed to 90°. Ask the patient to open & close their hands for 3 minutes. A positive test is indicated by reproduction of the patient's neurological / vascular symptoms. This is indicative of thoracic outlet syndrome. 3. **Adson's Test (Fig 7.2):** Palpate the patient's radial artery while they are sitting in a chair. Position their shoulder in approximately 45° of abduction & full external rotation, with full elbow extension. Ask the patient to look over the shoulder of the side being tested, extend their neck & hold their breath. Gently extend the arm from this position, in a continuous movement. A positive test is recorded as the radial pulse disappears. This is indicative of thoracic outlet syndrome.

COMPLETION	Interpretation
Lymphadenopathy	Check associated lymph nodes.
Distal Neurovascular Status	Full examinations required *(see relevant chapters)*. Particularly focus on pulses, dermatomes & myotomes, look for cervical myelopathy & auscultate for a subclavian artery murmur suggestive of mechanical obstruction.
QoL Impingement & Sleep	Asking patient about these helps to assess impact on life & therefore necessity for intervention.
Help Patient Dress	Good practice if patient has functional limitation.
Radiographs	Soft tissue / bony abnormalities.

FINISH:

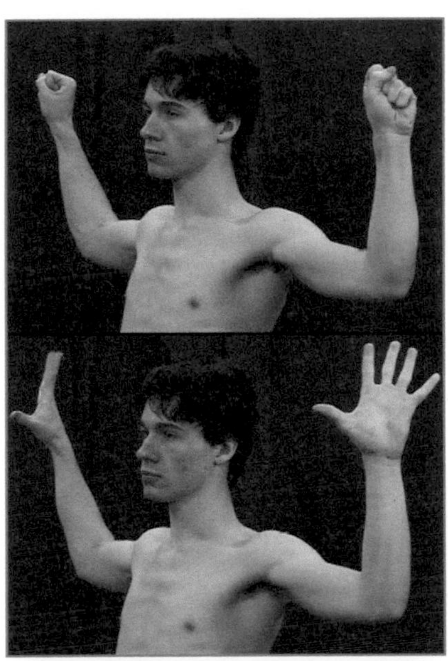

Fig 7.1: Roo's Test

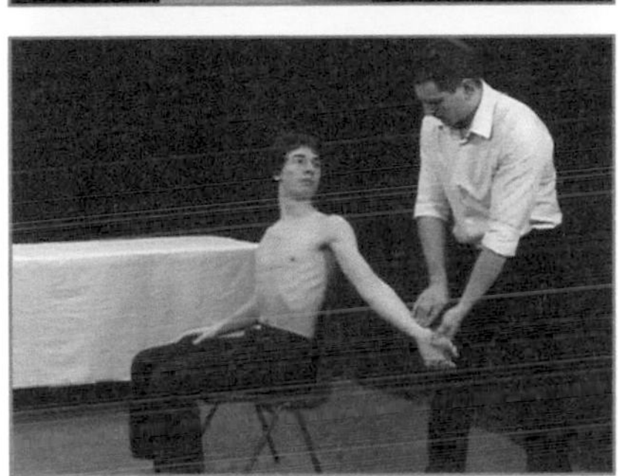

Fig 7.2: Adson's Test

SPINE EXAMINATION

START: Patient exposed to underwear.

First ask the patient to walk away a few steps, turn around & come back.

With the patient standing, inspect from FRONT, BACK & SIDES as follows:

LOOK	Interpretation
Scars	Post-operative e.g. discectomy (posterior midline), post-infective.
Swelling	Soft tissue / bony mass e.g. gibbus (fused vertebra causing abnormal protuberance at the thoracolumbar junction in TB / fracture).
Symmetry	Torticollis (involuntary neck contractions result in head tilting towards the side of the precipitating lesion / underlying pathology).
Deformity	• **Scoliosis:** May disappear with the patient sitting (secondary to leg length discrepancy) or persist (indicating a fixed / structural scoliosis). • **Kyphosis:** May disappear when the patient's shoulders are braced back (postural) or persist (fixed / structural). • **Lordosis:** May be obliterated e.g. OA, prolapsed IVD, ankylosing spondylitis. May be exaggerated e.g. spondylolisthesis, hip flexion deformity, exaggerated thoracic kyphosis.
Erythema	Inflammation.
Sinus	Post-operative, infective.
Muscle Wasting	Paraspinal muscles e.g. previous trauma, neurological or infection e.g. TB.

Ask about pain.

Feel for temperature changes with the back of your hand along the entire length of the spine.

FEEL	Interpretation
Pain	Systematically feel the bones, then soft tissues, starting from the top of the cervical spine, running down to the sacroiliac joints. Bony tenderness may indicate tumour / infection. Sacroiliac joint tenderness may indicate sacroiliitis e.g. ankylosing spondylitis. Paraspinal muscle tenderness may indicate mechanical back pain / spasm e.g. prolapsed IVD.
Stepping	Run fingers down midline of bony spine. An abnormal spinous process 'step' may indicate spondylolisthesis, fracture, tumour or infection.
Chest expansion	Ask the patient to breathe in, then out fully. Quickly place your thumbs (facing up) on the patient parasternally, then place your index fingers in the line of the 5th intercostal spaces. Ask the patient to take a deep breath in. Normal expansion = 5–7cm. This is grossly reduced in ankylosing spondylitis.

MOVE	Interpretation
Cervical Spine	• **Flexion** (80°) / **Extension** (50°) • **Lateral Flexion** (45°) • **Rotation** (80°) Repeat movements with downward pressure on head *(see orthopaedic neck examination).*
Thoracic Spine	• **Lateral Rotation:** With the patient sitting on the edge of a chair, arms on each ipsilateral hip, ask the patient to twist to each side. Normal = 40°.
Lumbar Spine	• **Forward Flexion:** Ask the patient to touch their toes with their legs straight & measure the distance from their fingertips to the floor. Normal = 7cm. This should also be tested using Schober's Test *(see special tests).* • **Extension:** Ask the patient to bend backwards. Normal = 30°. • **Lateral Flexion:** Ask the patient to slide their hand down the side of their leg. Normal = 30°.

SPECIAL TESTS	Interpretation
Schober's Test	Draw a line through both PSIS (Dimples of Venus). Mark the spine 5cm below & 10cm above this line. Keeping the tape measure in place, ask the patient to touch their toes & record the new distance between the outermost marks. Normal flexion = 5cm. This is reduced in lumbar spine pathology e.g. ankylosing spondylitis.
Lumbar Disc / Sciatic Nerve Pathology	The following tests assess nerve root compression (L4–S1). • **Bragard's Test:** Perform a straight leg raise on the patient, with the patient lying supine. Stop when back / leg pain or paraesthesia is precipitated. Now dorsiflex the foot, which will worsen symptoms (positive test). • **Lasègue's Test:** Following straight on from Bragard's Test, maintaining the angle of foot dorsiflexion. Flex the knee until pain is relieved, then further flex the hip, which will worsen symptoms (positive test). **Note: A free straight leg raise without restriction rules out disc / sciatic nerve pathology.**
Reverse Lasègue / Femoral Stretch Test	With the patient lying prone, flex the knee to 90° & lift the ankle superiorly, perpendicular to the couch. Back / thigh pain suggests femoral nerve root (L1–L4) compression.
Pelvic Compression	Push down gently on both ASIS, with the patient lying supine. Pain in the sacroiliac region suggests sacroiliitis e.g. ankylosing spondylitis.
Lhermitte's Sign	With the patient sitting in a chair, flex the cervical spine. Radicular pain indicates cervical nerve root compression e.g. spondylosis, prolapsed IVD.
Beevor's Sign	Place the patient's arms behind their head, whilst they are lying supine on the couch. Ask the patient to lift their head off the couch & observe the umbilicus. If the umbilicus moves to the side, there is weakness of the rectus on the opposite side, indicating T6–T12 spinal cord injury.
Abdominal Reflex	Gently swipe your finger around the umbilicus, imagining 4 quadrants. Failure of the umbilicus to twitch towards the stimulated quadrant indicates thoracic cord compression on that side. The nerve supply for the upper quadrant = T6–T10 & lower quadrant = T11–T12.

COMPLETION	Interpretation
Lymphadenopathy	Check associated lymph nodes.
Full Neurological Examination	This is required to fine tune the diagnostic level of pathology including: • **Cauda Equina:** Check for saddle anaesthesia, perianal sensation & anal tone (via a per rectum examination), which are decreased in cauda equine syndrome. • **Reflexes:** *See peripheral neurology.* • **Extensor Hallucis Longus:** Weakness suggests L5 nerve root pathology.
Full Vascular Examination	Rule out AAA as a cause of back pain. Assess vascular status of upper & lower limbs.
Waddell's Tests	5 categories of test help to rule out non-organic causes of back pain i.e. tenderness, simulation, distraction, regional disturbances & overreaction tests.
QoL Impingement & Sleep	Asking patient about these helps to assess impact on life & therefore necessity for intervention.
Help Patient Dress	Good practice if patient has functional limitation.
Radiographs	Soft tissue / bony abnormalities.

FINISH:

SHOULDER EXAMINATION

START: Patient exposure is ideally with blouse / shirt off. This is to assist the examination of the joint above (cervical spine) & below (elbow).

First ask the patient to walk away a few steps, turn around & come back, whilst checking for normal arm swing.

Remember to compare both sides throughout the examination.

Practice the elbow examination as a 'dance' in front of the mirror.

LOOK	Interpretation
Scapula Winging	Ask the patient to push their hands against a wall, with their elbows extended. Winging may be seen with a prominent medial scapula border. Lesions of the long thoracic nerve of Bell (C5–C7, innervates serratus anterior), may lead to winging.
With the patient sitting in a chair, examine the FRONT, SIDES, BACK, SUPERIOR joints & AXILLAE for:	
Scars	Traumatic or iatrogenic e.g. arthroscopy ports & post-operative scars.
Swelling	Look for soft tissue & bony swellings. Joint effusions present with swelling in the axilla. Apparent bony 'swellings' may indicate dislocation of the SCJ / ACJ. A swelling at the anterior-distal upper arm may represent a ruptured biceps tendon.
Symmetry	Check the alignment of the shoulder joint & associated muscle contour. This should be symmetrical. Significant asymmetry implies unilateral disease (or 1 shoulder is worse than the other). Symmetrical disease is associated with RA.
Deformity	Check for bony deformity, paying particular attention to the SCJ, clavicle & ACJ. SCJ & ACJ subluxation / dislocation may be more obvious from above. Shoulder dislocation may be present if the patient holds their arm in internal rotation (posterior dislocation) / external rotation (anterior dislocation).
Erythema	Inflammation e.g. RA.
Sinus	Post-operative, infective.
Muscle Wasting	Pectoral muscles (pectoral nerves), deltoid (shoulder contour is lost / square e.g. C5, axillary nerve lesion), trapezius (XI, accessory nerve), Supraspinatus (rotator cuff tear) & infraspinatus (C5–C6, suprascapular nerve lesion).

Ask about pain.

Feel for temperature changes with the back of your hand.

Systematically feel the shoulder joint, associated bony prominences & soft tissues.

FEEL	Interpretation
Pain	Start at the SCJ; feel along the line of the clavicle & around the ACJ. Feel around the glenohumeral joint & scapula. Feel trapezius, deltoid & infraspinatus. Extend the shoulder, feel supraspinatus & then the bicipital groove. The biceps tendon may be felt in this position by internally & externally rotating the humerus.
Axilla	The head of the humerus may be felt via the axilla. Also assess for lumps & lymphadenopathy.

Movements should ideally be tested actively & passively, with the patient standing.

Movements should be repeated with the scapula stabilised (pushing down on the shoulder).

Remember that shoulder ROM is particularly dependent on shoulder position.

MOVE	Interpretation
Abduction & External Rotation	Ask the patient to put their hands behind their head, pushing their elbows back. This is a good screening test for global active shoulder movement.
Adduction & Internal Rotation	Ask the patient to put their hands behind their back, thumbs pointing to the ceiling. The thumbs should normally reach T6. This is a good screening test for global active shoulder movement.
Abduction (coronal plane)	With the patient's arms by their sides, thumbs facing forward & elbows extended fully, ask the patient to fully abduct their arms. Supraspinatus initiates & is responsible for the first 0°–30° of abduction, deltoid is responsible for 30°–90° & the scapula-thoracic apparatus is responsible for the last 60° of abduction. Failure of abduction initiation may be due to supraspinatus tendinitis / rotator cuff tear. Painful arc syndrome represents pathology of the rotator cuff (this is usually due to compression of a chronically inflamed supraspinatus tendon, compressing against the acromion process resulting in pain between 60°–120° of abduction). Pain at the end of abduction (140°–180°) represents ACJ OA. Normal ROM = 0°–180°.
Flexion	Ask the patient to forward flex their shoulders, with their forearms fully pronated & elbows extended. Normal = 165° of flexion.
Extension	Ask the patient to extend their shoulders, with their forearms fully pronated & elbows extended. Normal = 60° of extension.
Adduction	Ask the patient to touch their opposite shoulder with each hand.
Internal Rotation	Ask the patient to internally rotate their shoulders, keeping their arms tucked into their sides (subscapularis). Normal = 60°–70° internal rotation (as the trunk prevents further movement). With the shoulder abducted to 90°, normal = 90° internal rotation. *Internal rotation may also be tested with the shoulder abducted & elbow flexed.*
External Rotation	Ask the patient to externally rotate their shoulders, keeping their arms tucked into their sides (infraspinatus & teres minor). Normal = 90°external rotation. *External rotation may also be tested with the shoulder abducted & elbow flexed.*

Muscle power is tested against resistance.

Remember to test muscle power 'like-for-like' where possible, comparing each side.

MUSCLE POWER	Interpretation
Supraspinatus	Resisted abduction 0°–30°. Position the patient's shoulder in 30° of forward flexion & 30° abduction, with the patient's forearm in full pronation (thumbs down). Test supraspinatus by asking the patient to 'push out' (abduct) against resistance.
Deltoid	Resisted abduction 30°–90°. Position the patient's shoulders in 90° of abduction, elbows fully flexed. Test deltoid by asking the patient to maintain this position against resistance.
Infraspinatus & Teres Minor	Resisted external rotation with elbows tucked into sides & flexed to 90°.
Gerber's Test	Position the patient's hand behind their back, with the dorsum of their hand touching their back & elbow flexed to 90°. Ask the patient to lift the dorsum of their hand off their back against mild resistance. If the patient is unable to do this or *'lift off'* even without resistance, this indicates **subscapularis** pathology.

SPECIAL TESTS	Interpretation
Multidirectional Instability	Ask the patient to lie supine at the edge of the couch, shoulder joint at the edge of the bed. Stabilise the scapula with one hand & test abnormal posterior / anterior movement of the humerus at the glenohumeral joint with your other hand. Instability implies capsule / ligament damage.
Apprehension-Relocation Test (Jobe's Test)	Ask the patient to lie supine on the examination couch, shoulder joint at the edge of the bed. Abduct the patient's shoulder to 90° & flex the elbow to 90°. Stabilise & feel the glenohumeral joint with one hand & externally rotate the joint with the other hand. Anterior instability is confirmed as the patient's face becomes 'apprehensive' due to pain (Apprehension Test). This pain may be relieved with the application of posterior (pushing down towards the couch) pressure to the shoulder (Relocation Test). This is positive for **anterior joint instability**. *It is best to avoid performing this test in the OSCE as it precipitates pain, so simply mention it instead.*
Neer's Test	Ask the patient to sit on the edge of the couch / in a chair. Internally rotate the patient's shoulder & pronate their forearm, keeping arms tucked by their sides. Stabilise the scapula & passively forward flex the shoulder in a continuous movement. If pain is reproduced, this is a positive test for rotator cuff impingement.

COMPLETION	Interpretation
Lymphadenopathy	Check associated lymph nodes.
Joint Above & Below	Full neck & elbow examination.
Distal Neurovascular Status	Full examinations required *(see relevant chapters)*. Particularly focus on pulses, dermatomes & myotomes. Axillary nerve (C5) sensation should be tested specifically over the lateral aspect of deltoid.
QoL Impingement & Sleep	Asking the patient about these helps to assess impact on life & therefore necessity for intervention.
Help Patient Dress	Good practice if the patient has functional limitation.
Radiographs	Soft tissue / bony abnormalities.

FINISH:

ELBOW EXAMINATION

START: Patient exposure is ideally with blouse / shirt off. This is to assist the examination of the joint above (shoulder) & below (wrist).

First look at the joint with the patient's arms alongside their body, in supination (palms forward). Comment on the carrying angle (normal 0°–15°).

Look at the joint with the patient's arms abducted to 90°, in supination (palms up).

Continue the examination, comparing both elbows, with the patient standing.

LOOK	Interpretation
Scars & Skin	Traumatic or iatrogenic e.g. arthroscopy ports & post-operative scars. Psoriasis patches on extensor aspects. Gouty tophi of joints (also check the pinna as tophi may occur here).
Swelling	Soft tissue e.g. RA, bone e.g. OA, bursa e.g. olecranon bursitis (student's elbow).
Symmetry	Check the alignment of the elbows & arms. This should be symmetrical. Significant asymmetry implies unilateral disease (or one elbow is worse than the other). Symmetrical disease is associated with RA.
Deformity	**Cubitus valgus** e.g. non-union of previous lateral condyle fracture, **cubitus varus** e.g. mal-union of previous supracondylar fracture in children, **ankylosis, flexion deformity.**
Erythema	Inflammation e.g. RA.
Sinus	Post-operative, infective.
Muscle Wasting	Wasting of arm & forearm muscles. Causes include previous trauma, neurological lesions or infection e.g. TB.

Ask about pain.

Feel for temperature changes with the back of your hand.

Systematically feel the elbow joint, associated bony prominences & soft tissues.

FEEL	Interpretation
Pain	This may be bony or soft tissue in origin, depending on anatomical location. Comment on the following common pathologies: • **Lateral Epicondylitis:** Tennis elbow. • **Medial Epicondylitis:** Golfer's elbow. • **Olecranon Bursitis:** Student's elbow.
Relation of Bony Prominences	The olecranon, medial & lateral epicondyles together form an inverted triangle that is best seen from behind. This triangle is altered in dislocation.
Joint Line	In particular, palpate the head of the radius, whilst pronating & supinating the patient's forearm. Feel for clicking if loose bodies are present within the joint.
Rheumatoid Nodules	Often present on the extensor surfaces of the arms / elbow joint.
Ulnar Nerve	Lies superficially, posterior to the medial epicondyle. May be 'rolled' under the fingers. Hypersensitivity may be due to e.g. ulnar neuritis / tardy ulnar palsy. Thickening may be due to e.g. leprosy.
Antecubital Fossa	Brachial artery, median nerve & biceps tendon.

Movements should ideally be tested actively, passively & against resistance.

Remember to test muscle power 'like-for-like' where possible, comparing each side.

MOVE	Interpretation
Ulnar-Humeral Joint	Ask the patient to extend & flex their elbow. Normal ROM = 0°– 140°.
Radio-Ulnar Joint	Ask the patient to flex their elbows to 90°, tucking them into their sides. Ask the patient to point their palms to the ceiling (supination) & then the floor (pronation). Normal ROM = 90° of pronation through to 90° of supination.
Locking	May occur with loose bodies in e.g. trauma, OA, osteochondritis dissecans.

COMPLETION	Interpretation
Lymphadenopathy	Check associated lymph nodes.
Joint Above & Below	Full shoulder & wrist examination.
Distal Neurovascular Status	Full examinations required *(see relevant chapters)*. Particularly focus on pulses, dermatomes & myotomes.
QoL Impingement & Sleep	Asking patient about these helps to assess impact on life & therefore necessity for intervention.
Help Patient Dress	Good practice if patient has functional limitation.
Radiographs	Soft tissue / bony abnormalities.

FINISH:

HIP EXAMINATION

START: Patient exposure to underwear. This is to assist examination of the joint above (spine) & below (knee).

First ask the patient to walk away a few steps, turn around & come back, to assess gait.

Comment on use of aids e.g. stick, frame, brace, shoes etc.

Perform Trendelenberg's Test *(see special tests)* first.

With the patient standing, inspect from the FRONT, BACK & SIDES of the joint.

LOOK	Interpretation
Scars	Traumatic or iatrogenic e.g. post-operative (anterior / posterior approach etc).
Swelling	Look for soft tissue & bony swelling e.g. lymphadenopathy, effusion (rare), tumour.
Symmetry	ASIS & greater trochanter levels should lie on a horizontal plane.
Deformity	Adduction / abduction (both may result in scoliosis), fixed flexion (may result in lordosis), leg length discrepancy (may result in scoliosis), rotational etc.
Erythema	Inflammation e.g. RA.
Sinus	Post-operative, infective e.g. TB.
Muscle Wasting	Gluteus, quadriceps etc.

Lay the patient on the couch supine.

Remember to examine the good side first.

Ask about pain.

Feel for temperature changes with the back of your hand.

FEEL	Interpretation
Pain	Systematically examine the hip: • **Greater Trochanter:** Palpated laterally (pain may suggest trochanteric bursitis). Also palpate the soft tissues around the greater trochanter. • **Femoral Head:** Lies deep to the femoral artery, at the mid-inguinal point. • **Adductor Longus:** Palpate medially along the entire length (adductor strain occurs in sports injury, adductor contracture occurs in OA). • **Ischial Tuberosity:** Palpated posteriorly (trauma). **Note: Turn the patient on their side to palpate the ischial tuberosities.**
Crepitus	Palpate for crepitus by rotating the hip medially & laterally. Crepitus suggests OA.
Lymphadenopathy	Assess inguinal lymph nodes.
Apparent Leg Length	Measure the distance from the xiphisternum to medial malleolus. Discrepancy indicates compensatory pelvic tilt, due to adduction / abduction deformity. **Note: Apparent length is longer for an abduction deformity & shorter for an adduction deformity.**
True Leg Length	Square the pelvis, aligning each ASIS in a horizontal plane. Demonstrate this by placing your elbow & hand (using the same upper limb) on each ASIS. Measure the distance from each ASIS to corresponding medial malleolus. Discrepancy indicates shortening of the affected limb. Isolate this to one of the following levels, first flexing the hips & knees to 90°, aligning the medial malleoli: • **Femoral Neck:** Place a thumb on each ASIS & middle finger on each greater trochanter. Imagine a line dropped vertically down from the ASIS & a 2nd line extended horizontally from the greater trochanter. Place your index finger at the point where these lines cross to form *Bryant's Triangle*. When the distance between the index & middle finger is shorter than the contralateral side, this indicates supratrochanteric shortening e.g. fracture, SCFE, Perthe's Disease, OA, DDH. • **Femoral Shaft:** Shortening is demonstrated as the knee of the affected limb lies proximal-inferior to the knee of the good limb e.g. fracture, infection. • **Tibia:** Shortening is demonstrated as the knee of the affected limb lies distal-inferior to the knee of the good limb e.g. fracture, infection.

Movements should ideally be tested actively, passively & against resistance, with the pelvis square.

Remember to compare each side, starting with the good side first.

Start with Thomas' Test *(see special tests)* to unmask fixed flexion deformity.

MOVE	Interpretation
Extension	Patient lies prone or on their side. Passively lifting the patient's leg may reveal 10° of normal hyperextension. In most hip pathologies, this is the first movement to be lost. Normal = 0°–10°. **Note: If Thomas's Test is positive, do not test extension.**
Flexion	Keeping the contralateral lower limb extended (back of thigh, calf & heel touching the couch = neutral position), flex the hip until the thigh touches the abdomen with the knee fully flexed, or until the pelvis starts moving. Normal = 150°.
Abduction	With the pelvis square, the angle of abduction is measured by drawing a vertical line distally from the ASIS. The angle subtended between this line & the long axis of the thigh is the angle of abduction. Normal = 45°. **Note: If there is an initial abduction deformity, measure true leg length by abducting the unaffected limb symmetrically to the affected limb.**
Adduction	With the pelvis square, the angle of adduction is measured by drawing a vertical line distally from the ASIS. The angle subtended between this line & the long axis of the thigh is the angle of adduction. Normal = 45°. **Note: If there is an initial adduction deformity, place the unaffected limb abducted off the side of the couch & adduct the affected limb in the horizontal plane, until the thumb appreciates movement of the ASIS.**
External & Internal Rotation	The hip & knee are flexed to 90°. Fix the knee with your left hand & secure the heel with your right hand. With the hip as a fulcrum, move the lower leg medially (normal external hip rotation = 30°) & laterally (normal internal hip rotation = 45°).

SPECIAL TESTS	Interpretation
Trendelenberg's Test (Fig 7.3)	***Perform at the start of the hip examination.*** This assesses stability. Stand opposite the patient & hold out your supinated hands. Ask the patient to place their hands (pronated) on yours. Perform the test on the good leg first, asking the patient to bend the knee of their affected leg. Normally, the weight bearing hip is held stable by the abductors & the pelvis rises on the unsupported side. If the weight-bearing hip is painful / unstable, the pelvis drops on the unsupported side (positive test) e.g. OA, abductor weakness, hip pain (all causes). **Note: You must anticipate that the patient may fall when standing on their affected hip & support them with your corresponding outstretched hand.**
Thomas's Test (Fig 7.4)	***Perform before testing movements.*** This unmasks a fixed flexion deformity. The patient should be lying flat on the couch. It may be easier to manipulate the patient kneeling down to the side of the couch. Place your left hand under the patient's lumbar spine. Ask the patient to flex both hips & knees fully (this will obliterate the normal lumbar lordosis). Perform the test on the good side first, asking the patient to hold their affected limb with both hands. With your other hand holding the lower leg / ankle, control full extension of the limb to be tested. Full extension is normally achieved with the lumbar lordosis still obliterated. If there is a fixed flexion deformity, the patient will arch their lumbar spine & the lumbar lordosis will reappear (pressure is relieved on your left hand). At the point where this occurs, bend the patient's knee such that their heel touches the couch & measure the angle between the couch & thigh = angle of flexion deformity.

COMPLETION	Interpretation
Lymphadenopathy	Check associated lymph nodes.
Joint Above & Below	Full spine & knee examination.
Distal Neurovascular Status	Full examinations required *(see relevant chapters)*. Particularly focus on pulses, dermatomes & myotomes.
QoL Impingement & Sleep	Asking patient about these helps to assess impact on life & therefore necessity for intervention.
Help Patient Dress	Good practice if patient has functional limitation.
Radiographs	Soft tissue / bony abnormalities.

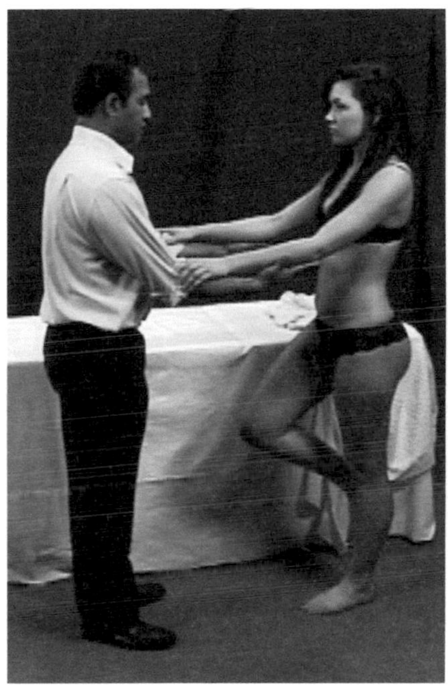

Fig 7.3: Trendelenberg's Test

Fig 7.4: Thomas's Test

FINISH:

KNEE EXAMINATION

START: Adequate patient exposure is ideally to underwear. This is to assist examination of gait, the spine, the joint above (hip) & below (ankle).

Comment on use of aids e.g. stick, frame, brace, shoes etc.

Ensure inspection from the FRONT, SIDES & BACK of the joint, comparing both knees with the patient standing.

LOOK	Interpretation
Scars	Traumatic or iatrogenic e.g. arthroscopy ports & post-operative scars. • **Anterior Midline Scar:** Total knee replacement. • **Suprapatellar Scar:** Quadriceps repair. • **Tibial Tubercle Scar:** Tubercle transfer for high riding patella / ACL surgery.
Swelling	• **Anterior:** Effusion, synovitis, prepatellar bursa, infrapatellar bursa. • **Lateral:** Meniscal cyst. • **Posterior:** Bakers cyst, popliteal aneurysm.
Symmetry	Check the alignment of the knees & legs. This should be symmetrical. Significant asymmetry implies unilateral disease (or one side is worse than the other). Symmetrical disease is associated with RA.
Deformity	Varus e.g. OA (measure interepicondylar distance, which will be increased). Valgus e.g. RA (measure intermalleolar distance which will be increased).
Erythema	Inflammation e.g. RA.
Sinus	Post-operative, infective.
Muscle Wasting	Check quadriceps VMO & calf muscles. Causes of muscle wasting include previous trauma, neurological lesions or infection e.g. TB.
With the patient on the examination couch, lying flat:	
Patella Tracking	Ask the patient to flex their knee to 90°. Tracking is confirmed as the patella moves in a J-shaped fashion (laterally in most cases) = tight vastus lateralis / patellofemoral ligament (PFL).

The remainder of the examination is also undertaken with the patient lying flat on the couch.

Ask about pain.

Feel for temperature changes with the back of your hand.

FEEL	Interpretation
Pain	Systematically examine the quadriceps, patella tendon, patella margins, knee joint margins & collateral ligaments. Pathology depends on site of pain & structural involvement e.g. lateral knee joint margin (meniscus), tibial tuberosity (Osgood Schlatter's Disease), patella tendon (tendinitis).
Continuity	Check continuity of the extensor apparatus.
Quadriceps	Measure the circumference of quadriceps bilaterally. Choose a fixed point e.g. 10cm above the superior border of the patella.
Effusion	• **Cross-Fluctuation Test:** Empty the medial compartment superiorly, then empty the suprapatellar pouch inferiorly, then compress the lateral compartment. Look for fluid transmission across the joint, appearing medially. • **Patellar Tap Test:** Empty the suprapatellar pouch inferiorly & then with the index finger of your other hand, push the patella downward, onto the femur. A spring back is positive. This is for moderate effusions. • **Bulge Test:** Empty the medial compartment superiorly & then compress the lateral compartment. Look for a bulge in the medial compartment. This is for minimal effusions.
Synovial Thickening	Try lifting the patella between your thumb & index finger. It will not be possible with a thickened synovium e.g. RA / TB synovitis.
Flexion Deformity	Place your hand under the patient's knee & ask them to push the back of their knee down to the couch. If your hand is compressed, there is no flexion deformity. If there is a gap under the patient's knee when they perform this manoeuvre, without hand compression, there is a flexion deformity. Flexion deformities may be classified as follows: • **Correctable:** Passive downward pressure corrects the deformity e.g. extensor lag. • **Fixed:** Passive downward pressure does not correct the deformity.

Movements should ideally be tested actively, passively & against resistance.

Remember to compare each side.

MOVE	Interpretation
Extension	Normal = 0°. Passively lifting the patient's leg may reveal 10° of normal hyperextension. >10° hyperextension = genu recurvatum.
Flexion	Normal = 150°.
Crepitus	Feel for crepitus with your hand over the patella-femoral junction at the same time as flexing & extending the knee e.g. trauma, OA.
Straight Leg Raise	Ask the patient to lift their leg off the bed, keeping their knee extended. If this is not possible, there may be extensor apparatus damage or a flexion deformity.

It may be more efficient to perform special tests in the following order:

SPECIAL TESTS	Interpretation
Posterior Sag Sign	Square the patient's legs with 90° knee flexion. Maintaining this position, flex the hips to 90°, supporting the lower legs from below, placing an arm underneath & in line with the ankles. The test is positive when the tibia of the affected knee sags towards the examination couch, indicating **posterior cruciate ligament rupture**. This is clearly seen as the prominence of the tibial tuberosity, usually visible in the lower leg, becomes obliterated. It is important to assess posterior sag prior to performing Lachman's test, as if it is missed, a false positive Lachman's Test may be elicited.
Posterior Drawer Test	Square the patient's legs with their knees flexed to 90°. Explain to the patient that you are going to sit on their foot, check that they have no pain, gain permission & sit on the patient's feet. Grasp the upper tibia firmly, thumbs placed on the anterior joint line & apply posterior pressure. Significant posterior glide is positive for a **posterior cruciate ligament rupture**.
Lachman's Test	Performed with 20–30° knee flexion, with the patient's heel on the couch. Stabilise the patient's thigh with one hand & pull the tibia anteriorly with your other hand (thumb on joint line, hand behind calf). The test is positive if there is anterior tibial translation. This indicates an **anterior cruciate ligament rupture**. **Continue straight on to testing the collateral ligaments as you are in a position that facilitates easier assessment already.**
Collateral Ligaments	Test the collateral ligaments with 30° knee flexion. Tuck the patient's foot under your arm & stabilise their knee on either side of the joint with both hands. Use a combination of body movement & pressure on the knee to apply valgus (testing the medial collateral ligament) & varus stress (testing the lateral collateral ligament). Springiness with a firm endpoint is normally felt. Absence of an endpoint is positive for a collateral ligament rupture. Repeat collateral ligament tests with 0° knee extension. Valgus / varus deviation in 0° knee extension is always abnormal.
McMurray's Test	Place the thumb & index finger of one hand along the joint line to detect any 'clicks' & pain that is positive for a meniscus tear. Fully FLEX the leg, then in one smooth motion EXTEND the knee joint (by moving the patient's lower leg with your other hand). To test each meniscus, the following leg orientations are required throughout extension to open up the joint line: • **Medial Meniscus:** Foot external rotation & lower leg abduction (valgus) (throughout extension). • **Lateral Meniscus:** Foot internal rotation & lower leg adduction (varus) (throughout extension).
Patella Tests	• **Friction Test:** Move the patella superiorly & inferiorly, pressing it down against the femur. Painful grating is experienced if the central portion of articular cartilage is damaged. • **Zolen's / Clark's Test:** Press the patella down against the femur & ask the patient to contract their quadriceps. Pain is suggestive of patellofemoral OA. • **Apprehension Test:** Displacing the patella laterally with the thumb, whilst gently flexing the knee may induce pain & anxiety. This is a positive test & the patient will resist further movement. Diagnostic of recurrent patella subluxation / dislocation.

COMPLETION	Interpretation
Lymphadenopathy	Check associated lymph nodes.
Joint Above & Below	Full examination of the ankle & hip required *(see relevant sections)*.
Distal Neurovascular Status	Full examinations required *(see relevant chapters)*. Particularly focus on pulses, dermatomes & myotomes.
QoL Impingement & Sleep	Asking patient about these helps to assess impact on life & therefore necessity for intervention.
Help Patient Dress	Good practice if patient has functional limitation.
Radiographs	Soft tissue / bony abnormalities.

FINISH:

ANKLE & FOOT EXAMINATION

START: Patient exposure is ideally with trousers / skirt off.

Check the patient's shoes for pattern of wear.

First ask the patient to walk away a few steps, turn around & come back.

MUSCLES & TENDONS	Interpretation
Plantarflexors	Ask the patient to walk on their tip-toes.
Dorsiflexors	Ask the patient to walk on their heels.
Inverters	Ask the patient to stand on the outside edges of their feet.
Everters	Ask the patient to stand on the inside edges of their feet.

Remember to compare both sides throughout the examination.

Look at the ankle & foot with the patient standing, then sitting in a chair.

With the patient standing, look at the 3 x foot arches (medial / lateral / transverse).

With the patient sitting, look between the toes for ulcers, corns or callosities.

Do not forget to look at the plantar surface of the foot.

LOOK	Interpretation
Scars	Traumatic or iatrogenic e.g. post-operative.
Swelling	Look for soft tissue & bony swelling that may be traumatic, inflammatory or systemic. Suspect systemic cause with bilateral ankle oedema.
Symmetry	Asymmetrical callosities imply uneven distribution of load.
Deformity	Previous fracture, short / ruptured Achilles tendon, talipes (club foot), pes planus (flat foot), hallux valgus, mallet toe (DIPJ flexion deformity), hammer toe (PIPJ deformity), claw toes (DIPJ & PIPJ deformity), overriding toes. Most deformities are exaggerated on weight bearing.
Erythema	Inflammation e.g. RA.
Sinus	Post-operative, infective.
Muscle Wasting	Check the anterior, posterior & lateral compartments of the lower leg.

The patient should already be sitting in a chair.

Ask about pain.

Feel for temperature changes with the back of your hand.

FEEL	Interpretation
Pain	**Soft Tissues:** Achilles tendon (may palpate defect in rupture), peroneal tendons (behind lateral malleolus), dorsiflexion tendons, medial foot ligaments e.g. deltoid, lateral foot ligaments e.g. bifurcate, plantar fascia (plantar fasciitis). **Bones:** Palpate each joint individually. Check for malleolar tenderness. Squeeze the metatarsophalangeal joints (RA). Individually assess the remaining small bones of the feet.
Capillary Refill	Normal = 2–3 seconds.

MOVE	Interpretation
Ankle Joint	Grasp the lower leg with your left hand & hold the heel with your right hand. Assess dorsiflexion (normal = 15°) & plantar flexion (normal = 55°). Movements may be painful & restricted in arthritis or absent with arthrodesis.
Subtalar Joint	Grasp the lower leg with your left hand & hold the heel with your right hand. Assess inversion & eversion (normal = 15°). Movements may be painful & restricted in arthritis.
Midtarsal Joint	Grasp the heel with your left hand & hold the mid-foot with your right hand. Assess inversion & eversion (normal =15°).
Toes	Ask the patient to curl & extend their toes. Test the hallux individually & against resistance.

SPECIAL TESTS	Interpretation
Tenosynovitis	**Flexors / Inverters:** Palpate along the tendons behind the medial malleolus. Milk out synovial fluid from the tendons by running fingers proximally along them. **Tibialis Posterior:** Plantarflexion & eversion of the foot will precipitate pain just posterior to the medial malleolus. Check for gaps that indicate rupture e.g. RA & pes planus. **Peroneal:** Plantarflexion & inversion of the foot will precipitate pain behind the lateral malleolus. Now ask the patient to evert against resistance & feel for 'snapping' of a thickened, inflamed peroneal tendon.
Thompson's Test	Position the patient prone with their feet off the edge of the couch. Squeezing the calf should cause plantar flexion of the ankle. If not, this is pathognomonic of a ruptured Achilles tendon.
Tinel's Tarsal Tunnel Test	Percuss the posterior tibial nerve as it runs through the tarsal tunnel. This is located posterior to the medial malleolus. Reproduction of symptoms suggests tarsal tunnel syndrome.

COMPLETION	Interpretation
Lymphadenopathy	Check associated lymph nodes.
Joint Above & Below	Full knee examination. There is no joint below!
Distal Neurovascular Status	Full examinations required *(see relevant chapters)*. Particularly focus on pulses, dermatomes & myotomes. Glove in stocking distribution of paraesthesia / anaesthesia is suggestive of DM.
QoL Impingement & Sleep	Asking patient about these helps to assess impact on life & therefore necessity for intervention.
Help Patient Dress	Good practice if patient has functional limitation.
Radiographs	Soft tissue / bony abnormalities.

FINISH:

OSCE QUESTIONS

Gait

Q: What are the different phases of a normal gait?

Phase	Notes

Stance	• The foot is in contact with the ground during the stance phase.
	• The stance phase represents 60% of the gait cycle when walking.
	• The stance phase may be further classified as follows:
	  • **Heel Strike**: The heel hits the floor.
	  • **Foot Flat:** The whole of the foot makes contact with the floor.
	  • **Mid Stance:** Weight is transferred from the heel to the front of the foot.
	  • **Toe-Off**: Pushing off with the toes for forward propulsion.

Swing	• The swing phase represents 40% of the gait cycle when walking. • The foot swings forward (to become the leading foot again) & the contralateral leg supports the body.
Note: During walking there is a **'double stance'** period when both feet are in contact with the ground. When running, the stance phase becomes progressively shorter until a point is reached when neither foot is in contact with the ground, the so-called **'flight phase'**.	

Q: What different types of gait do you know of?

Gait	Notes
Antalgic	Decreased stance & increased swing phase on the affected leg (due to pain).
Cerebellar	Broad based 'drunkard' gait (cerebellar ataxia).
High Stepping	Due to foot drop (common peroneal nerve damage).
Parkinsonian	Shuffling 'festinant' gait.
Short Leg	The affected hip appears to dip (congenital, iatrogenic, previous fracture).
Spastic	Jerky & scissoring (upper motor neuron lesion).
Trendelenberg	The patient lurches over the side of the bad hip to compensate for 'abductor weakness'. Causes of abductor weakness include OA, DDH, neuromuscular disorders & trauma.

Osteoarthritis (OA)

Q: What is osteoarthritis?

This is a disease of synovial joints, characterised by cartilaginous loss & bony response, resulting in joint degeneration & destruction. OA is the most common joint disease worldwide.

Q: What are the causes of osteoarthritis?

Cause	Explanation / Examples
Primary	No underlying cause is attributable to joint degeneration. Chronic degeneration of joints occurs with age.
Secondary	An underlying cause is attributable to joint degeneration. These may be classified as follows: • **Congenital:** Perthe's Disease / SUFE • **Endocrine:** Acromegaly • **Infective:** Osteomyelitis • **Inflammatory:** RA • **Metabolic:** Diabetes / Gout • **Nutritional:** Obesity • **Traumatic:** Iatrogenic / Accidental • **Other:** Paget's Disease of Bone / SLE

Q: What are the clinical features of osteoarthritis?

Features	Explanation
Pain	• Sharp ache / burning sensation. • Worse with movement. • Worse at the end of the day.
Stiffness	• Worse at the end of the day. • Decreased range of motion due to pain / joint destruction.
Loss of Function	• Due to bony response e.g. osteophytes, Heberden's (DIPJ) & Bouchard's (PIPJ) Nodes. • Due to deformity e.g. valgus / varus.

Q: How would you make a diagnosis of osteoarthritis?

Diagnosis involves taking a **full history** & performing a **thorough clinical examination**. No laboratory or pathological tests are useful. Diagnosis is confirmed by radiological features as follows (Fig 7.5):

Memory: 'LOSS' for the radiological features of OA.

Loss of Joint Space (or narrowing)

Osteophyte Formation

Subchondral Sclerosis

Subchondral Cysts

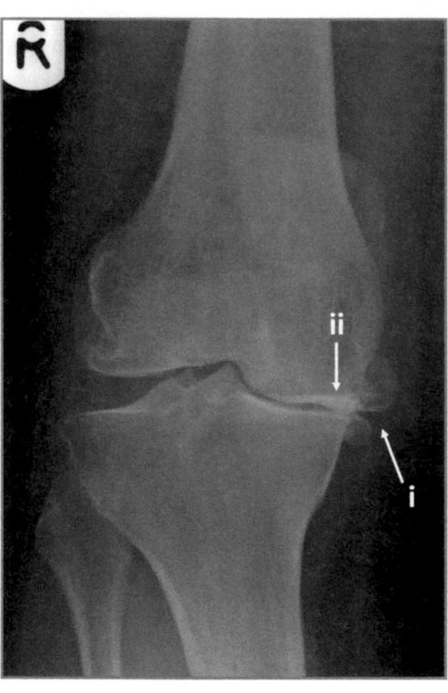

Fig 7.5: AP radiograph illustrating osteoarthritis of the right knee. Most pathology is seen at the medial joint line with loss of joint space, osteophytes (i) & subchondral sclerosis (ii) present.

Q: What are the treatment options for osteoarthritis?

These may be classified as follows:

Conservative	Medical	Surgical
Aids e.g. Walking Stick	Analgesic Ladder	Osteotomy (realign)
Lifestyle Modification	Intra-Articular Corticosteroids (if there is a superadded inflammatory component)	Arthroplasty (replace)
OT / PT		Arthrodesis (fuse)
Patient Education		

Rheumatoid Arthritis (RA)

Q: What is rheumatoid arthritis?

A chronic, systemic inflammatory disorder, with an autoimmune component, that primarily affects joints (polyarthritis) in a symmetrical pattern. The characteristic pathology includes chronic synovitis, polyarthritis, joint deformity & ankylosis. RA affects <1% of the population & is 4 times more common in women.

Q: What are the clinical features of rheumatoid arthritis?

The hallmark feature of RA is a symmetrical polyarthritis & joint deformity. Clinical features may be classified as intra- / extra-articular as follows:

Intra-Articular	Interpretation
Pain	Due to synovitis & worse with movement. The joint may be warm & tender.
Swelling	Due to localised inflammation & joint effusions.
Stiffness	Characteristic early morning stiffness (>1 hour) or after prolonged inactivity.
Loss of Function	Due to joint swelling & destruction.
Deformity	Many deformities exist e.g. valgus, varus, subluxation, ulnar deviation of the MCPJs, radial deviation of the wrist (Fig 7.6), Z-thumb, swan neck, boutonniere (Figs 8.1–8.3), CMCJ subluxation, atlanto-axial joint subluxation.
Extra-Articular	**Interpretation**
Skin	Rheumatoid nodules, erythema nodosum, pyoderma gangrenosum, palmar erythema.
Cardiovascular	Myocarditis, pericardial effusion, pericarditis, vasculitis.
Eyes	Keratoconjunctivitis sicca, episcleritis, uveitis.
Kidneys	Chronic inflammation causing amyloidosis, damage due to treatment (Gold, NSAIDs).
Lungs	Fibrosis due to disease or treatment, effusions, nodules (Caplan Syndrome).
Neurological	Carpal tunnel syndrome.
Felty's Syndrome	RA associated with splenomegaly, anaemia, neutropaenia, thrombocytopaenia & lymphadenopathy.

Q: How would you make a diagnosis of rheumatoid arthritis?

After taking a **full history** (including family history & association with EBV) & performing a **thorough clinical examination**, I would consider the following:

Diagnosis	Interpretation
Blood Tests	• FBC, U&Es, CRP, ESR. • Rheumatoid Factor (positive in 80%). • HLA–DR4.
X-Ray	Changes may be: • **Early:** No change or soft tissue swelling & loss of joint space. • **Late:** Bony erosions, severe joint destruction & subluxation.
American College of Rheumatology Criteria (1987)	4 criteria must be met to diagnose RA: • Morning stiffness >1 hour on most mornings for ≥6 weeks. • Arthritis & soft-tissue swelling of ≥3 joint groups, for ≥6 weeks. • Arthritis of hand joints, present for ≥6 weeks. • Symmetrical arthritis, present for ≥6 weeks. • Subcutaneous nodules in specific places. • Rheumatoid factor at a level >95th percentile. • Radiological changes suggestive of joint erosion. **Note: Treatment should be started prior to meeting criteria, as early treatment is associated with decreased joint erosion.**

Q: What is this radiograph & what are points A & B?

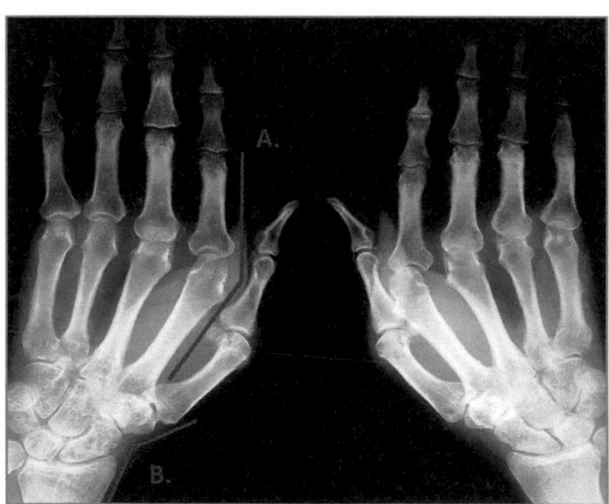

Fig 7.6: Radiograph of the hands, with characteristic features of rheumatoid arthritis.

A: Ulnar deviation of the metacarpophalangeal joints (MCPJ).

B: Radial deviation of the wrist.

Q: What is the management of rheumatoid arthritis?

Conservative	Medical	Surgical
Aids e.g. Walking Stick	Analgesic Ladder	Osteotomy (realign)
Lifestyle Modification	Corticosteroids	Arthroplasty (replace)
OT / PT	Disease Modifying Anti-Rheumatic Drugs (DMARDS) e.g. Gold, Penicillamine	Arthrodesis (fuse)
Patient Education		Tendon Transfer
	TNFα Inhibitors	Synovectomy

Ankylosing Spondylitis (AS)

Q: What is ankylosing spondylitis?

An inflammatory disorder from the group of seronegative spondylarthropathies. Progressive inflammation typically affects the vertebral column & sacroiliac joints, leading to bony ankylosis (fusion). Ankylosing spondylitis is 3 times more common in males & presents around the age of 25 years. The annual incidence is 7/100,000 & it is associated with HLA-B27.

Q: What are the clinical features of ankylosing spondylitis?

Intra-Articular	Interpretation
Back Pain	Low back pain that is worse in the morning. Other joints may be affected e.g. hips & knees. Sacroiliitis may also be present & painful.
Stiffness	Back & joint stiffness, characteristically worse early in the morning. Early morning stiffness may gradually ease with activity.
Loss of Function	Limitation of spinal movement due to bony ankylosis. Lateral flexion is commonly 1st to be affected.
Enthesitis	Inflammation of a tendon, ligament or joint capsule insertion point into bone.
Fractures	More common in patients with ankylosing spondylitis.
Osteoporosis	More common in patients with ankylosing spondylitis.
Other	Increased thoracic kyphosis, loss of lumbar lordosis, chest expansion <5cm.
Extra-Articular	**Interpretation**
Cardiovascular	Aortitis, conduction defects, myocarditis.
Eyes	Anterior uveitis (most common & affects 20%), iritis.
Lungs	Apical pulmonary fibrosis.
Neurological	Cauda equina syndrome.

Q: How would you make a diagnosis of ankylosing spondylitis?

Diagnosis depends on taking a **full history** & performing a **thorough clinical examination**. There are no laboratory or pathological tests available to diagnose ankylosing spondylitis, however the following investigations should be considered:

Investigations	Interpretation
Blood Tests	• FBC, CRP, ESR. • Rheumatoid factor (negative). • HLA-B27 (positive in 90% of patients).
Spine X-Ray	• Intervertebral disc ossification. • Bamboo spine (syndesmophytes are bony bridges that span the intervertebral joints, giving it the appearance of bamboo) (Fig 7.7). • Sacroiliac joint fusion (Fig 7.8).
CT / MRI	• May show early signs of sacroiliitis.

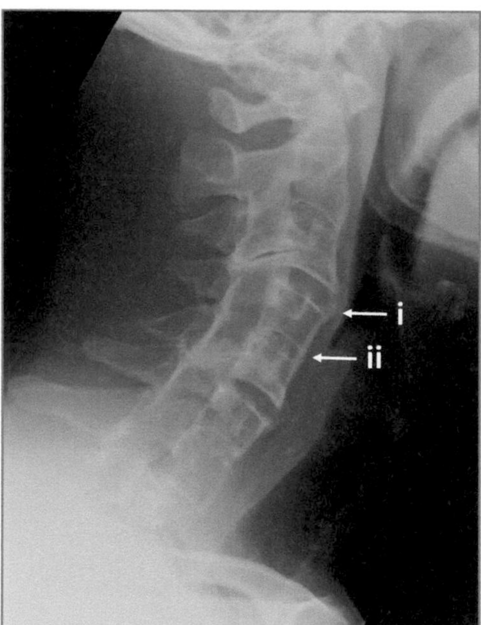

Fig 7.7: Lateral cervical spine radiograph of a patient with ankylosing spondylitis. Bamboo spine, with syndesmophytes (i) & vertebral fusion (ankylosis) (ii) present.

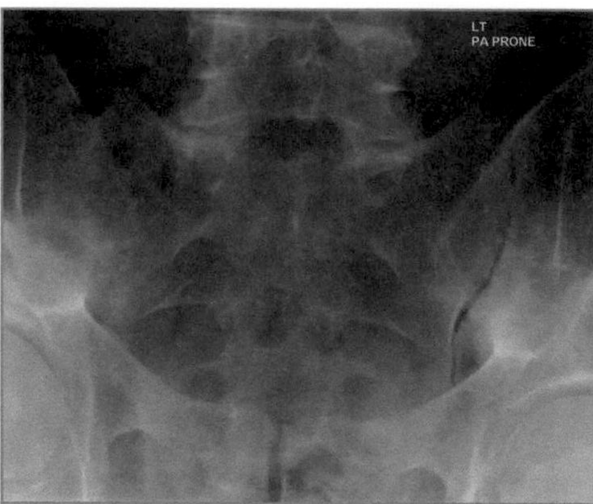

Fig 7.8: PA radiograph of the pelvis in a patient with ankylosing spondylitis. Sacroiliac joint fusion is visible on the right side when compared with the left, where the joint line is clearly visible.

Q: What are the treatment options for ankylosing spondylitis?

Conservative	Medical	Surgical
Aids e.g. Walking Stick	Analgesic Ladder	Osteotomy (realign)
Lifestyle Modification	Corticosteroid Injections	Arthroplasty (replace)
OT / PT	TNFα Antagonists	Arthrodesis (fuse)
Patient Education		

Paget's Disease of Bone

Q: What is Paget's Disease?

Paget's Disease (also known as osteitis deformans) is a chronic condition of bone involving mixed osteoclast & osteoblast activity. It is the 2nd most prevalent metabolic bone disease, commonly affecting middle-aged / elderly populations. The aetiology is largely unknown, however environmental, genetic & viral factors have been suggested. There are 3 distinct phases:

Phase	Notes
Osteolytic	Characterised by enhanced bone resorption due to osteoclast activity. This results in discrete lytic lesions of affected bone (Fig 7.9).
Mixed	Osteoblasts also become active & lay woven bone. The result is disorganised bone formation.
Osteosclerotic	Osteoclast & osteoblast activity decline. Resulting in abnormal, eroded & sclerotic bone.

Note: Paget also described Paget's Disease of the nipple.

Q: What does the following radiograph show?

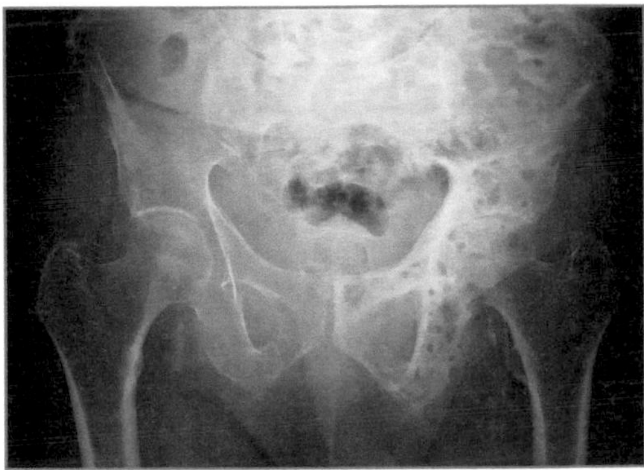

Fig 7.9: Paget's Disease of the left hip.

This is a radiograph of the pelvis. There is a mixed lytic & sclerotic picture, with:

- **Lytic lesions** affecting the left hemi-pelvis & femoral head.
- **Bony sclerosis** of the left acetabulum region.

The most likely diagnosis is Paget's Disease of the left hip.

Q: What are the clinical features of Paget's Disease?

Paget's Disease is usually asymptomatic. Clinical features are related to the extent & phase of disease, including the presence or absence of complications. They include:

Features	Examples
Symptoms	• **Bone Pain** (due to microfractures). • **Muscle Weakness** (due to disuse / pain). • **Neurological Symptoms** e.g. deafness (due to cranial nerve VIII compression) / trigeminal neuralgia (due to cranial nerve V compression).
Signs	• **Bony Deformity & Enlargement.** • **Localised Pain.** • **Skin Erythema & Warmth** (due to vascular response). • **Gait Abnormalities** (due to bony deformity / pain).
Complications	• **Bony:** Deformity, OA & pathological fractures. • **Cardiovascular:** High output cardiac failure (due to increased vascularity). • **Endocrine:** Secondary hyperparathyroidism may develop in 10% of patients. • **Metabolic:** Hypercalcaemia (due to prolongued immobility). • **Neurological:** Focal neurological deficits & neuropathic pain (due to spinal cord / cranial nerve / peripheral nerve compression). • **Neoplastic:** Osteosarcoma may develop in 1% of patients. • **Social:** Immobility.

Q: What specific investigations would assist your diagnosis of Paget's Disease?

After taking a **full history** & performing a **thorough clinical examination,** I would consider the following specific tests in addition to those ordered as part of a comprehensive work up:

Investigation	Interpretation
Blood Tests	• **Alkaline Phosphatase:** Raised with increased osteoblastic activity & reflects disease extent. • **Calcium:** Usually normal. May be raised with prolonged immobility. • **Phosphate:** Normal. • **TFT:** Thyroid function tests rule out secondary hyperparathyroidism.
Urine Tests	• **Urinary Hydroxyproline:** Raised with increased osteoblastic activity (it is a collagen breakdown product).
Radiology	• **X-ray:** Lytic lesions in early disease (Fig 7.5). Thickened, eroded & sclerotic bone in late disease. Bony enlargement, with increased radiodensity & trabeculations is pathognomonic. • **CT / MRI:** Helpful to assess complications including joint involvement, articular abnormailities & spinal cord involvement. • **Bone Scan:** Helpful to assess disease extent.

Q: What is the management of Paget's Disease?

Conservative	Medical	Surgical
Aids e.g. Walking Stick	Analgesic Ladder	Repair Fractures
OT / PT	Bisphosponates	Osteotomy (realign joint)
Hot / Cold Packs	(decrease bone turnover)	Arthroplasty (replace joint)
Massage	Calcitonin	Nerve / Spinal Cord Decompression
Patient Education		Tumour Resection / Amputation

Painful Shoulder

Q: What is the differential diagnosis of a painful shoulder?

Pathology	Example
Soft Tissues	Adhesive capsulitis (frozen shoulder), rotator cuff injury / rupture, supraspinatus tendinitis, subacromial bursitis, long head of biceps tendinitis, suprascapular nerve entrapment.
Joint	Acromioclavicular OA, glenohumeral OA, recurrent dislocation, subluxation.
Bone	Infection, neoplasm.
Referred Pain	Cervical spondylosis, cardiac ischaemia.

Q: What is adhesive capsulitis (frozen shoulder)?

An idiopathic condition characterised by decreased ROM & chronic pain. Active & passive ROM becomes limited in all directions, however external rotation is usually worst affected. Adhesions gradually form until the glenohumeral joint is stiff & only scapular-thoracic movement remains. Diagnosis is based on a full history & thorough clinical examination, although other causes of shoulder pathology must be ruled out e.g. infection / rotator cuff injury.

Q: What is the management of adhesive capsulitis?

Conservative	Medical	Surgical
Physiotherapy	Analgesic Ladder	Manipulation Under Anaesthetic
	NSAIDs	Arthroscopic Release
	Corticosteroid Injection	

Q: What is shoulder impingement syndrome?

Impingement of the supraspinatus tendon passing throught the subacromial space causing inflammation of the tendon, eventually leading to its rupture. This condition also is known as the painful arc syndrome.

Features	Examples
Symptoms	• Painful shoulder (overhead activity). • The painful arc (60°–120° abduction). • Limited range of movements. • Weakness.
Signs	• Impingement testing (Neer's Test, Hawkin's Test, Jobe's Test).
Causes	• Trauma (can cause complete rupture of tendon). • Idiopathic. • Bony spur (from OA of ACJ or under surface of acromium). • Subacromial bursal pathology.

Diagnosis	• **Clinical investigation:** Injection of local anaesthetic into the subachromial space, relieves pain during clinical examination, hence assisting in diagnosis.
	• **Radiological diagnosis**:
	  • **X-ray:** May show a calcified tendon or bony spur in the subacromial space.
	  • **MRI:** Delineates rotator cuff muscle pathology (including rupture).

Complications	• Inflammation can lead to tendon rupture. • Instability of shoulder. • Poor shoulder function.

Q: What is the treatment of Impingement syndrome?

Conservative	Medical	Surgical
PT (strength)	Analgesic Ladder	Subacromial Decompression +/- ACJ Excision
Limit Impingement Position Activity	Steroid Injection	Rotator Cuff Repair (arthroscopic or open)

Ankle & Foot Pathology

Q: Can you briefly explain the following conditions: Achilles tendon rupture, claw toes, hallux rigidus & valgus, hammer toes & talipes equinovarus?

Condition	Explanation
Achilles Tendon Rupture	Inability to plantar flex foot due to rupture.
Claw Toes	Flexion deformity of PIPJ & DIPJ with compensatory hyperextension of MTPJ.
Hallux Rigidus	Degenerative joint disease of big toe MTPJ causing joint pain & stiffness.
Hallux Valgus	Prominence of 1st metatarsal head (the most common foot deformity). This may be associated with valgus deviation of the great toe.
Hammer Toes	Flexion deformity of PIPJ with compensatory DIPJ extension.
Talipes Equinovarus (club foot)	Plantar flexion, inversion, adduction deformity of the foot, with the heel in varus. The foot appears 'clubbed'.

Q: What is the pathophysiology of these conditions?

Condition	Explanation
Achilles Tendon Rupture	Spontaneous or traumatic (direct injury). Sudden plantar flexion (forced) causes tendon rupture. Spontaneous ruptures are associated with an increased risk of future contralateral rupture.
Claw Toes	Usually seen in neurological disorders e.g. poliomyelitis & peroneal muscle atrophy (Charcot-Marie-Tooth Disease). Also seen in RA.
Hallux Rigidus	Osteoarthritis of 1st MTPJ (either primary or secondary).
Hallux Valgus	Underlying deformity is forefoot splaying (metatarsus primus varus).
Hammer Toes	Caused by imbalance between extrinsic & intrinsic muscles causing fixed PIPJ flexion.
Talipes Equinovarus (club foot)	Most common congenital foot deformity.

Q: What operative treatment might you consider for these conditions?

All these conditions can be treated conservatively & medically e.g. appropriate footwear & analgesic ladder. Specific operative treatments for the various conditions are as follows:

Condition	Operative Treatment
Achilles Tendon Rupture	***Non-Operative:*** Serial Casts (in equinus, semi-equinus & neutral positions). ***Operative:*** Open / Percutaneous Repair & Cast Immobilisation.
Claw Toes	Tendon Transfer (long toe flexor to extensors), Joint Excision, Arthrodesis.
Hallux Rigidus	Silastic Joint Replacement, Arthrodesis.
Hallux Valgus	Bunionectomy & Realignment Osteotomy (Scarf, Akin, Chevron, Wilson's, Mitchell's).
Hammer Toes	Tendon Transfer, Joint Excision, Arthrodesis.
Talipes Equinovarus (club foot)	Plaster / Wedging / Splinting (Ponseti), Surgical Correction e.g. Percutaneous Tibialis Anterior Lengthening.

CHAPTER 8
HANDS

K Asaad
BH Miranda
M Nicolaou
SK Al-Ghazal

CHAPTER CONTENTS

Hand Examination

OSCE Questions

- Dupuytren's Disease
- Ganglion
- Trigger Finger

HAND EXAMINATION

START: Patient sitting opposite you, with hands resting on a table / supported by a pillow.

Expose patient above the elbows bilaterally.

Look for any aids e.g. splints.

LOOK	Interpretation
Scars	Trauma, post-operative e.g. carpal tunnel release, tendon repair.
Swelling	Soft tissue or bony mass. Describe *6 x S's* as for any lump *(see lumps 'n' bumps chapter).*
Symmetry	Symmetrical disease is associated with RA.
Deformity	Dupuytren's contracture, nerve lesions (*see upper limb nerves chapter),* OA, RA**.**
Erythema	Inflammation, infection.
Sinus	Post-operative, infective.
Muscle Wasting	Thenar / hypothenar eminences, dorsal intermetacarpal wasting (Fig 11.4).
Other	• Raynaud's Phenomenon. • Onycholysis (nail separation from the nail bed e.g. psoriasis). • Gangrene. • Check elbows for psoriatic plaques.

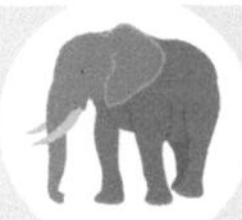

Memory: Look for features of OA & RA specifically

OA	RA
Heberden's Nodes (bony DIPJ swelling)	**Rheumatoid Nodules** (Fig 8.1) (25% of patients with RA have rheumatoid nodules)
Bouchard's Nodes (bony PIPJ swelling)	**Boutonniere Deformity** (Fig 8.2) (PIPJ flexion & DIPJ hyperextension)
Thumb Squaring (1st CMCJ subluxation)	**Swan-Neck Deformity** (Fig 8.3) (PIPJ hyperextension & DIPJ flexion)
	Z-Thumb (MCPJ extension & IPJ flexion)
	Radial Deviation of the Wrist (Fig 7.6)
	Ulnar Deviation of the Digits (Fig 7.6) (capsular loosening & ligamentous laxity of the MCPJ)

Ask about pain.

Feel for temperature changes (dorsal & ventral) with the back of your hand.

FEEL	Interpretation
Capillary Refill	Gently press fingertip for 5 seconds then observe time for colour to change from white to pink. Normal = 2–3 seconds.
Dupuytren's Contracture	Feel for palmar fascia thickening & look for associated Garrod's Pads (Figs 8.4 & 8.5).
Rheumatoid Nodules	Subcutaneous lesions, usually on extensor surfaces.
Tenderness	Palpate each joint separately & systematically. Check the anatomical snuffbox for tenderness that may be associated with a scaphoid fracture, particularly in the acute setting.
Hand Nerves	Screen for the following nerve injuries, by assessing fine touch. If an injury is suspected, perform a thorough nerve examination *(see upper limb nerves)*: • **Radial Nerve:** (1st dorsal web space). • **Median Nerve:** (thenar eminence). • **Ulnar Nerve:** (palmar aspect of little finger).

Remember to test like-for-like.

MOVE	Interpretation
Global Functional Assessment	• Flex thumb. • Make a fist & fan out fingers. • Abduct & adduct fingers. • Demonstrate opposition. • Power grip.
Range of Motion	• Both active & passive range of motion should be recorded. • Prayer sign (normal = 70° wrist extension). • Reverse prayer sign (normal = 90° wrist flexion). • Radial deviation (normal = 20° wrist radial deviation). • Ulnar deviation (normal = 50° wrist ulnar deviation). • Pronation / supination (normal = 85° / 80°).

MOVE	Interpretation
Digital Tendons	*Thumb:* • **Abductor pollicis brevis** (against resistance). • **Flexor pollicis longus** (against resistance). • **Extensor pollicis longus** (patient keeps palmar surface of hand flat on a table & lifts thumb). *Digital Flexors:* • **Flexor digitorum profundus** (against resistance). • **Flexor digitorum superficialis** (against resistance). *Digital Extensors:* • **Extensor digitorum communis** (against resistance). • **Extensor indicis & extensor digiti minimi** (tested together by asking the patient to make a fist & extend their index & little fingers – 'Bullhorns').

SPECIAL TESTS	Interpretation	
Tinnel's Test	Take the patient's hand, palmar surface up. Tap their forearm, proximal to distal, along the course of the median nerve (warn the patient that you are going to do this). Ensure that tapping is extended over the region of the carpal tunnel, which may reproduce carpal tunnel syndrome symptoms e.g. tingling.	
Phalen's Test	Ask the patient to hold their wrists in complete & forced flexion (similar to the reverse prayer sign), pushing the dorsal surfaces of both hands together for 1 minute. This compresses the median nerve as it runs through the carpal tunnel, such that reproduction of carpal tunnel syndrome symptoms may occur.	
Finkelstein's Test	Positive for De Quervian's Tenosynovitis. Pain & inflammation of the extensor pollicis brevis & abductor pollicis longus tendons, may be reproduced / exacerbated by asking the patient to flex their thumb, form a fist over it, then ulnar deviate their wrist.	
Fine Functional Assessment	Pick up a key (pincer grip). Unbutton & button shirt. Pick up a pen & write a short sentence.	
Two-Point Discrimination Test	Normal:	<6mm.
	Fair:	6–10mm.
	Poor:	11–16mm.
	Protective:	1 point perceived.
	Anaesthetic:	No points perceived.

FINISH	Interpretation
Lymphadenopathy	Check associated lymph nodes.
Joints	Full examination of the wrist & elbow is required (joints above).
Upper Limb Neurovascular Status	Full examinations required (see relevant sections). Particularly focus on pulses, dermatomes & myotomes.
QoL Impingement & Sleep	Asking patient about these helps to assess impact on life & therefore necessity for intervention.
Help Patient Dress	Good practice if patient has functional limitation.
Radiographs	Soft tissue / bony abnormalities.

FINISH:

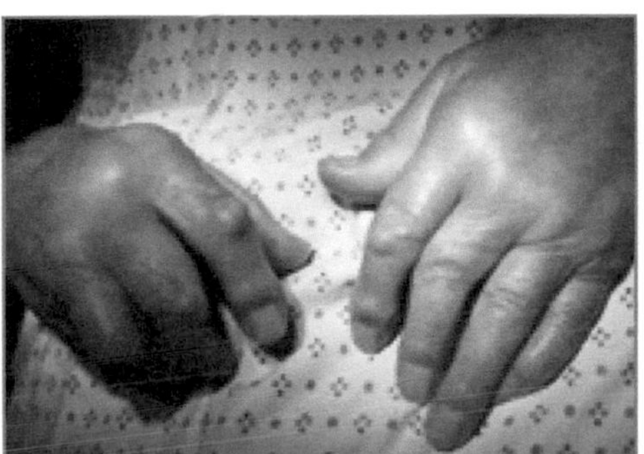

Fig 8.1: Rheumatoid Nodules. Symmetrical polyarthropathy of the hands with rheumatoid nodules visible on the extensor surfaces of the digits.

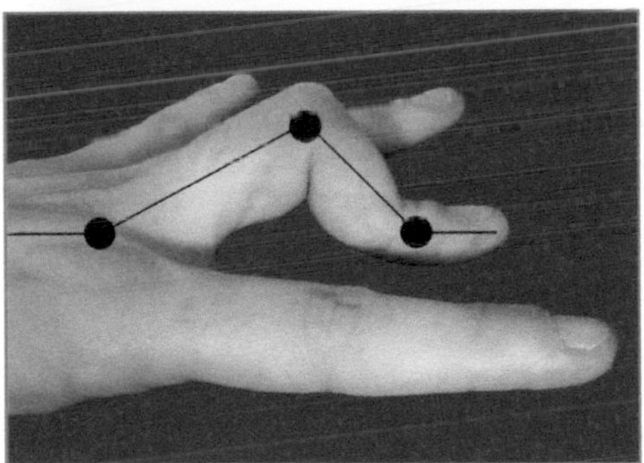

Fig 8.2: Boutonniere's Deformity of the left middle finger. There is PIPJ flexion with DIPJ hyperextension.

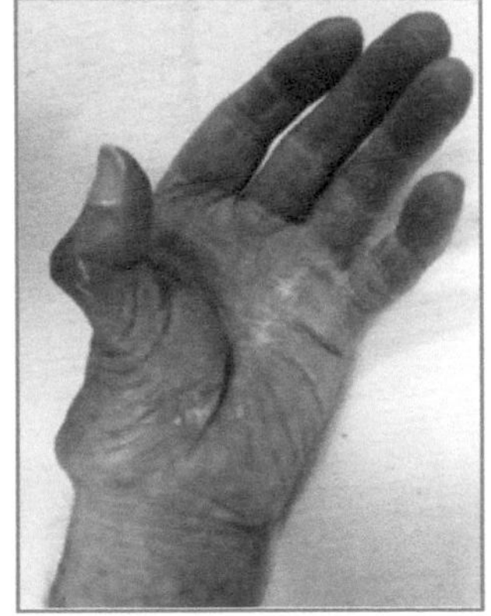

Fig 8.3: Z-Thumb Deformity. Left Z-thumb deformity in a patient with rheumatoid arthritis.

OSCE QUESTIONS

Dupuytren's Disease

Q: What is Dupuytren's Disease?

This is a fibrotic disease of the palmar & digital fascia (superficial & deep) characterised by subcutaneous nodules, cords & flexion contractures (Fig 8.4).

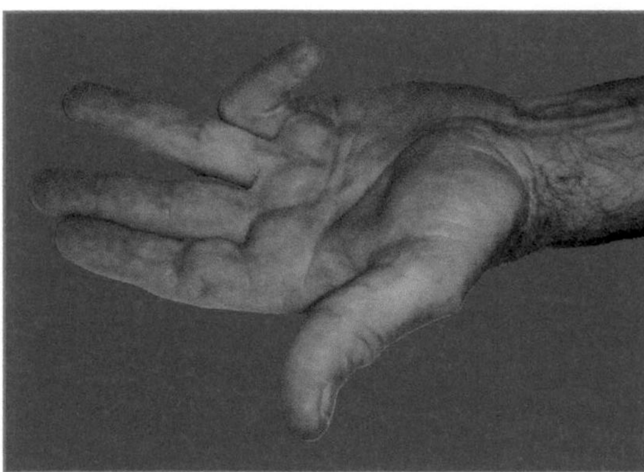

Fig 8.4: Dupuytren's Disease affecting left hand. Note the flexion contracture of the little finger PIPJ, with palmar fascia thickening.

Q: What are the risk factors?

Congenital	Acquired
Genetic e.g. Caucasians of Celtic / Northern European Origin	Age >50
Male: Female = 10:1	Smoking
Diabetes	Epilepsy (possibly anti-epileptic medication)
	Infection
	Manual Labour (evidence is equivocal)

Q: Where else would you look for associated conditions?

Location	Description
Dorsal PIPJ	Garrod's Pads (Fig 8.5).
Plantar Surface of Foot	Ledderhose's Disease (fibrosis of the plantar fascia).
Penis	Peyronie's Disease (fibrotic plaques of the corpus cavernosa & tunica albuginea).

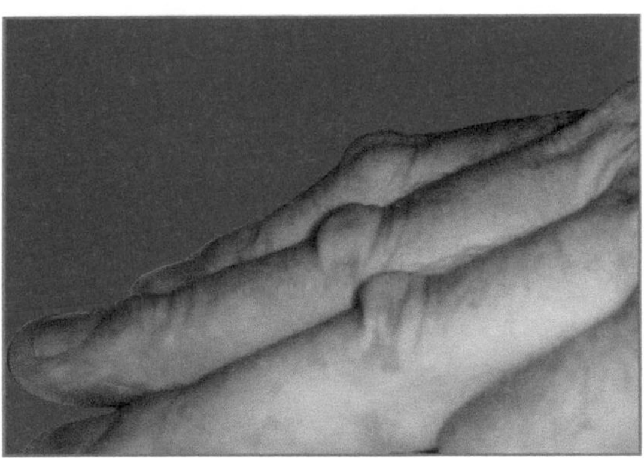

Fig 8.5: Garrod's Pads. These present as thickenings of the dorsal surfaces of the PIPJs.

Q: What are the indications for surgery?

- Pain & increasing disability.
- Any PIPJ & MCPJ joint flexion contracture >30°.

Q: What are the options for surgery?

This depends on the patient's co-morbidities, wishes & functional demands on the hand. Options include:

Surgical Option	Notes
Fasciotomy	Division of the diseased cord.
Fasciectomy	Excision of diseased fascia.
Dermatofasciectomy	Excision of diseased fascia & overlying skin (may require a skin graft).
Amputation	Considered in severe cases.

Q: What are the complications of surgery?

Immediate	Early	Late
Neurovascular Damage	Haematoma	Recurrence (50% at 10 years)
	Infection	Incomplete Joint Release
	Skin Flap Necrosis	Wound Breakdown
		CRPS
		Scar Contracture

Ganglion

Q: What is a ganglion?

- A mucinous filled cyst commonly located near a joint / tendon.
- It may communicate with the joint itself.
- It is the most common benign soft tissue tumour of the hand.

Q: What are the common sites for ganglia?

- **70% on the dorsal wrist.**
- **20% on the volar wrist.**
- **10% other sites:** Dorsal DIPJ (known as mucous cysts).
  Flexor sheath.
  PIPJ.

Q: What investigations would assist your diagnosis of a ganglion?

Diagnosis centres primarily on taking a **full history** & performing a **thorough clinical examination**. Investigations to consider include:

Investigation	Notes
X-Ray	Rule out co-existing degenerative joint disease.
USS	Inexpensive & non-invasive method of visualisation. Differentiates solid from liquid lesions.
MRI	For more detailed visualisation of extent.

Q: What are the treatment options?

Conservative	Interventional	Surgical
Patient Education & Monitoring	Aspiration +/- Steroid Injection (high risk of recurrence)	Excision (open or arthroscopic)

Trigger Finger

Q: What is a trigger finger?

Difficulty extending the finger from a flexed position. The finger may catch (or trigger) during motion or lock in the flexed position. It may be primary or congenital. It is associated with diabetes, carpal tunnel syndrome, De Quervain's Tenosynovitis, hypothyroidism, rheumatoid arthritis, renal disease & amyloidosis.

Q: Can you describe the arrangement of tendon sheath?

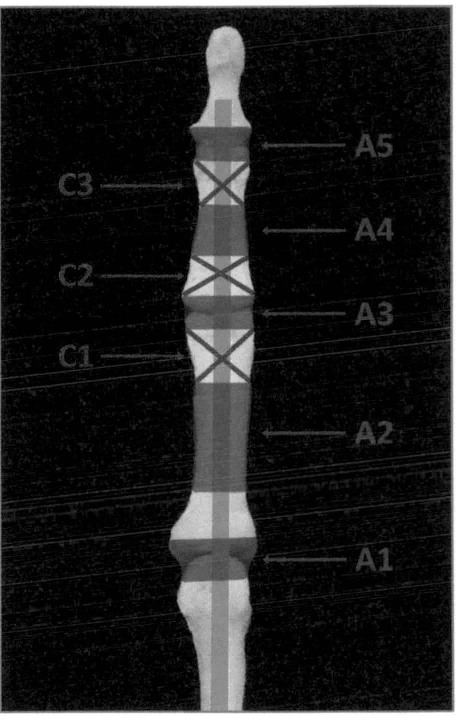

Fig 8.4: Diagrammatic representation of the flexor tendon sheath, illustrating:

Line of Flexor Tendons (FDP & FDS)

Annular Pulleys (A1–A5)

Cruciate Pulleys (C1–C3)

- The FDS & FDP tendons glide under a complex pulley system to enable the PIPJs & DIPJs to bend.
- There are 5 annular pulleys (A1–A5). A1 is the most proximal, located approximately at the level of the MCPJ. The A3 & A5 pulleys are located approximately at the level of the PIPJ & DIPJ respectively. The A2 & A4 pulleys are located at the shaft of the proximal & middle phalanges respectively.
- There are 3 cruciate pulleys (C1–C3). These alternate between the A2–A5 pulleys.

Q: What is the mechanism of triggering?

- Pathological narrowing of the tendon sheath tightens the gliding space for the tendons.
- Increased friction causes inflammation & further space reduction.
- The tendon may then catch or become stuck at the annular pulley (A1).

Q: What are the treatment options?

Conservative	Medical	Surgical
Patient Education & Monitoring.	Steroid Injection of Tendon Sheath.	Surgical Division of A1 Pulley.
Behaviour Modification e.g. Night Time Splinting (for adults).		

CHAPTER 9
VASCULAR

M Singh
J Lorains
K Asaad
DJA Scott

CHAPTER CONTENTS

Peripheral Arterial Examination

Varicose Veins Examination

OSCE Questions

- Arterial Insufficiency
- Abdominal Aortic Aneurysm
- Thoracic Outlet Syndrome
- Raynaud's Syndrome
- Carotid Artery Stenosis
- Deep Vein Thrombosis
- Deep Venous Insufficiency & Venous Hypertension
- Varicose Veins
- Gangrene

PERIPHERAL ARTERIAL EXAMINATION

START: Patient lying on bed, with shirt unbuttoned / off & legs exposed.

INSPECTION	Interpretation
Memory: **SNUGGS**	
Skin	**Hands:** Tar staining, wasting of small muscles of the hand (a rare finding in thoracic outlet syndrome). **Face:** Xanthelasma, corneal arcus. **Abdomen:** Obvious pulsatile mass. **Legs:** Discolouration (due to haemosiderin deposition), shiny skin.
Nails	Tar staining, onycholysis, thick & brittle.
Ulcers	Malleoli & pressure areas. Check between toes. Lift the lower limbs to check the heels & underneath the legs. Remember to describe any ulcer BEDS *(see lumps 'n' bumps chapter).*
Guttering & Gangrene	Venous guttering, gangrene (Fig 9.1), tissue loss.
Scars	Amputations (Fig 9.2), scars from previous surgery (cephalic & basilic vein harvesting scars from bypass procedures may be present on the arms).

Ask about pain.

Examine each side comparing both upper & lower limbs.

Examine the good side first.

PALPATION	Interpretation
Memory: **PC BOAT**	
Pulses	Radial, brachial, carotid, feel for AAA, femoral, popliteal, DP & TP. Note presence of any aneurysms & describe as for any other lump *(see lumps 'n' bumps chapter).*
Capillary Refill	Test the capillary refill time in the upper & lower limbs until blanching occurs, then release. Normal reperfusion occurs over 2–3 seconds. **Note: Capillary refill time may be affected by conditions other than PAD.**
Buerger's Angle & Test	Gently raise each leg & note the angle at which pallor occurs. In a normal subject pallor should not develop, even with 90° of leg elevation. Pallor developing with ≤20° leg elevation indicates severe peripheral arterial disease. Also note any venous guttering. Buerger's Test is then performed by swinging the leg down over the side of the bed & looking for reactive hyperaemia indicative of peripheral arterial disease (positive test). This should be repeated on the contralateral limb.The Pole test can also be used, which involves the application of a Doppler probe to the toe, then elevating the leg & measuring the height at which the Doppler signal disappears by means of a calibrated pole.
Oedema	DVT, lymphoedema, post-surgical.
Allen's Test	This assesses ulnar & radial arterial supply to the hand. Occlude both arteries, then ask the patient to repeatedly open & close their hand until it becomes pale. Release the artery to be tested & note the time for reperfusion. Repeat for the other artery. The ulnar artery is usually dominant.
Temperature	Feel for temperature changes by running the back of your hand proximally to distally over limb.

AUSCULTATION	Interpretation
Memory: CALF	
Bruits	Listen for arterial bruits, indicative of turbulent flow: • **C**arotid • **A**orta • I**L**iac • **F**emoral

COMPLETION	Interpretation
ABPI	Measure BP at the brachial artery. Using a hand-held Doppler, measure the BP at the DP & TP, then divide the highest ankle BP by the highest brachial BP. If resting ABPI is normal, get the patient to do 10 heel toe raises & re-check the ABPI.
VV Examination	Can have mixed arterial & venous disease.
Cardiac Examination	Full cardiac examination & ECG.
Neurological Examination	Full neurological examination e.g. diabetic neuropathy may be present.
BP & HR	Hypertension & AF common.
Investigations	Order appropriate investigations including Duplex, MRA, CTA, IADSA.

FINISH:

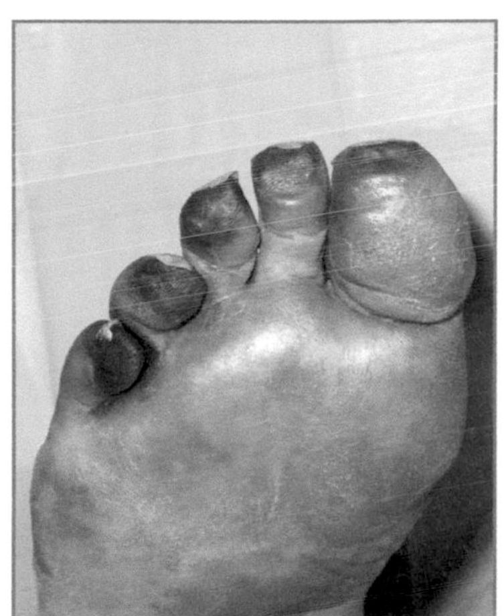

Fig 9.1: Right foot (plantar view) of a patient with peripheral arterial disease. The forefoot appears dusky & there are black, dry areas on the toes indicative of gangrene.

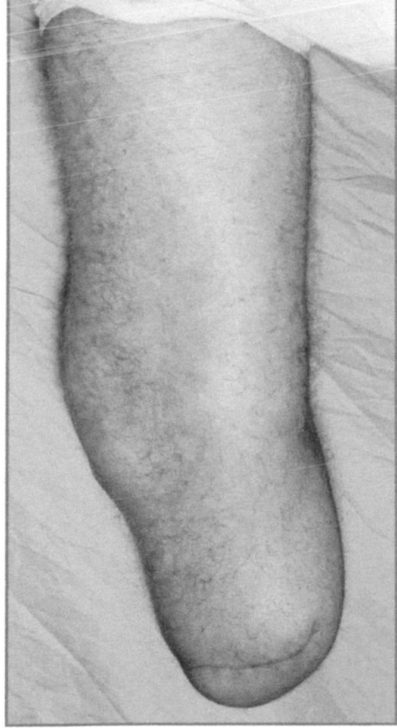

Fig 9.2: Right below knee amputation. Note the flap formed from the skin & muscles of the posterior compartment.

VARICOSE VEINS EXAMINATION

START: Patient initially standing, exposed to underwear.

INSPECTION	Interpretation
6 x S's	Describe dilated tortuous varicose veins as for any other lump (Fig 9.3) *(see lumps 'n' bumps chapter).* **Note: Varicosities above the SPJ relate to the LSV, but those that are below the SPJ may relate to either the LSV or SSV.**
Skin	Venous eczema, haemosiderin deposition, lipodermatosclerosis. Note the gaiter area especially.
Oedema	Could be secondary to DVT or lymphoedema.
Ulcers	LSV distribution is usually over the medial malleolus. SSV distribution is usually over the lateral malleolus. Remember to describe any ulcer BEDS *(see lumps 'n' bumps chapter).*
Scars	Groin crease scar e.g. high tie & LSV stripping. Popliteal fossa scar e.g. SPJ ligation surgery. Small scars along leg e.g. stab avulsions.

Ask about pain.

Examine each side comparing one limb to the other.

Examine the good side first.

PALPATION	Interpretation
SEC FFP TR	Assess compressible dilated tortuous varicose veins as for any other lump *(see lumps 'n' bumps chapter).*
Saphena Varix	Palpate over the SFJ for a saphena varix. This lies 4cm below & lateral to the pubic tubercle & is a smooth, soft bluish swelling that disappears on lying down.
Cough / Tap Test*	Palpate VV distally & tap proximally or ask the patient to cough. A transmitted impulse distally suggests incompetent valves proximal to the point of palpation.
Trendelenberg Test*	Patient lying down. Empty veins by milking proximally. Place pressure over SFJ & ask patient to stand up. If control is achieved then possible SFJ incompetence exists.
Tourniquet Test*	Patient lying down. Empty veins by milking proximally. Place tourniquet proximally around thigh & ask patient to stand up. If control is achieved then the level of incompetence is at / above the tourniquet level. If not, then move the tourniquet down the thigh & repeat until control is achieved.
Perthe's Test*	Once control has been achieved by the tourniquet test, ensure the patient is standing & ask them to move up & down on tip toes. If veins distend or the patient experiences pain, this suggests an incompetent deep venous system & therefore a LSV strip may worsen symptoms.

***Note: These clinical tests have now been superseded by hand-held Doppler & portable Duplex scanning & have little place in current practice.**

Hand-Held Doppler	With patient standing, place Doppler over the SPJ. Squeeze the calf & listen for Doppler sound. One whoosh with abrupt cut-off suggests a competent valve. If followed by a second whoosh this suggests reflux. Repeat by listening over the SFJ. Currently most vascular surgeons will use a portable Duplex scanner to assess varicose veins.

AUSCULTATION	Interpretation
Bruits	Listen over the femoral arteries for bruits, there may be an AVF e.g. post-femoral artery catheterisation / IVDUs.

COMPLETION	Interpretation
Full Abdominal Examination	Including PR examination for any masses that may cause venous obstruction.
ABPI	Influences the use of compression stockings for varicose veins: ABPI >1.3 – Avoid compression stockings due to calcified vessels. ABPI between 0.8 & 1.3 – Safe to use compression. ABPI between 0.5 & 0.8 – Only light (Class I) compression stockings to be used. ABPI <0.5 – Avoid compression as may compromise arterial blood supply.
Investigations	Order appropriate investigations including Duplex scan, MRV.

FINISH:

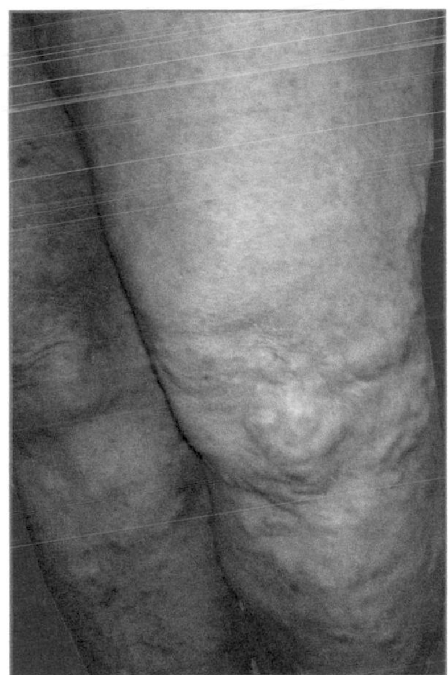

Fig 9.3: Bilateral varicose veins in a 54-year-old lady. There are multiple bluish, dilated & tortuous varicosties on the thigh & lower legs bilaterally. The limbs are oedematous & there are some venous telangiectasia present.

OSCE QUESTIONS

Arterial Insufficiency

Q: What are the symptoms & signs of acute arterial insufficiency?

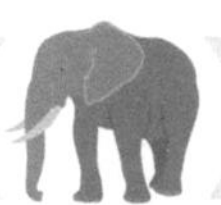

Memory: The 6 x P's of acute arterial insufficiency:

Symptom/Sign	Notes
Pain	Acute/sudden onset of pain in the affected limb.
Paraesthesia	Presence of a pins & needles sensation.
Pallor	Pale appearance.
Pulselessness	Loss of distal pulses in comparison to opposite limb.
Paresis	Motor weakness progressing to paralysis.
Perishingly Cold	Cold on palpation.

Q: What is the Fontaine Classification?

Grade	Description
I	Asymptomatic.
IIA	Intermittent claudication walking >200m & no rest pain.
IIB	Intermittent claudication walking <200m & no rest pain.
III	Rest / nocturnal pain.
IV	Gangrene / necrosis.

Q: What is the significance of the ABPI?

- An ABPI ≤0.9 may be used as a haemodynamic marker of PAD
- ABPI measurements relate to the severity of chronic ischaemia as follows:

ABPI	Notes
>1.3	Abnormal vessel hardening e.g. arterial calcification due to diabetes.
0.9-1.3	Normal range.
0.5-0.9	Moderate arterial disease.
<0.5	Severe arterial disease.

Q: What is critical limb ischaemia?

- Chronic ischaemic rest pain or the presence of ischaemic skin lesions (ulcers or gangrene).
- The term *'critical limb ischaemia'* only applies to chronic ischaemic disease (Fontaine Classification Grade III / IV), lasting >2 weeks.
- Some papers further classify this into:

i) **Subcritical Ischaemia:** Rest pain + ankle pressure >40mmHg.

ii) **Critical Ischaemia:** Rest pain + tissue loss/ankle pressure <40mmHg.

Abdominal Aortic Aneurysms (AAA)

Q: What is an abdominal aortic aneurysm?

Abnormal dilation of the abdominal aorta by >50% of its normal diameter (Fig 9.4).

Q: What are the clinical features of AAA?

Classification	Clinical Features
Asymptomatic	Most are asymptomatic & diagnosed incidentally on ultrasound.
Mass	Pulsatile abdominal mass.
Compression	Early satiety, nausea, vomiting, urinary tract symptoms & venous thrombosis.
Erosion	Back pain due to erosion into adjacent vertebrae.
Embolisation	Ischemic toes.
Rupture	Hypovolaemic shock & sudden death.

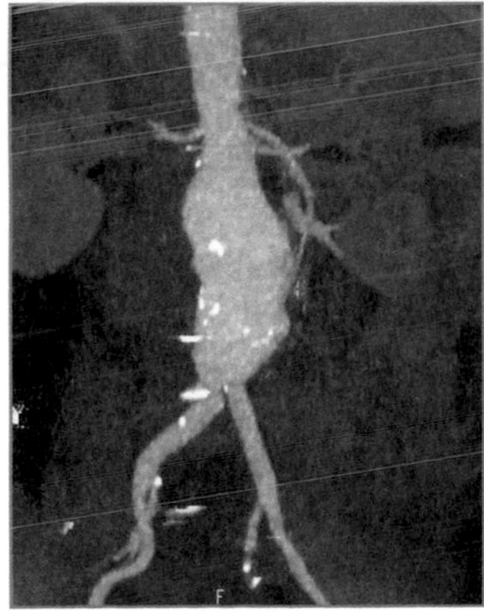

Fig 9.4: Aortic Aneurysm CT Reconstruction:

Sagittal CT reconstruction of a large abdominal aortic aneurysm.

Q: What is the risk of rupture of an AAA?

Risk of rupture is related to diameter as follows:

AAA Diameter	Rupture Risk (per annum)
<5.5cm	<1%
5–5.6 cm	10%
6–6.5 cm	20%
6.5–7 cm	25%
7–8 cm	33%
>8 cm	>50%

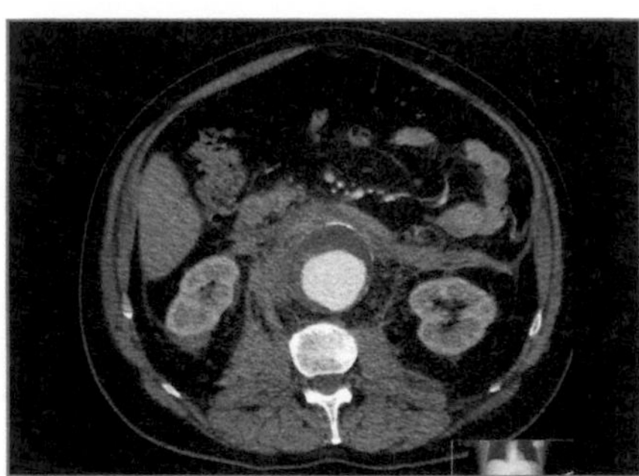

Fig 9.5: Ruptured AAA CT.

Contrast enhanced CT scan illustrating a ruptured abdominal aortic aneurysm. The contrast is high density in the aorta, which is surrounded by thrombus & a high density calcified wall. There is mixed density fluid surrounding the aorta consistent with rupture of the aneurysm.

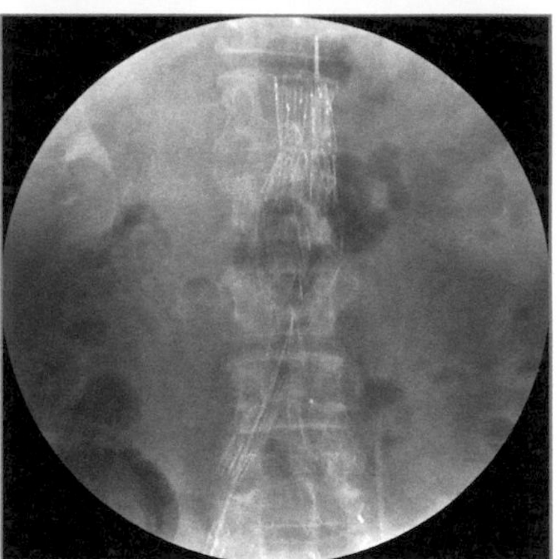

Fig 9.6: EVAR Radiograph.

Endovascular aneurysm repair (EVAR) of an abdominal aortic aneurysm.

Q: What is the elective management of a AAA?

Management depends on AAA diameter:

Diameter	Management
<3cm	No aneurysm.
3–4.4cm	Annual USS monitoring.
4.5–5.4cm	3-monthly monitoring offered.
>5.5cm	Referral to vascular surgeon. Patient offered elective repair (open repair or EVAR if possible). (Fig 9.6)

Q. What are the indications for AAA repair?

- Symptomatic patient
- Diameter >5.5cm
- Diameter increasing by 1cm per annum

Thoracic Outlet Syndrome

Q: What is thoracic outlet syndrome?

- A syndrome describing the symptoms & signs caused by arterial, venous or nerve compression as these major structures pass between the clavicle & 1st rib.

Q: What are the causes of thoracic outlet syndrome?

Cause	Example
Congenital	Cervical rib.
Acquired	Pathological enlargement of the 1st rib. Scalenus muscle hypertrophy. Fractured clavicle.

Q: What are the clinical features of thoracic outlet syndrome?

Clinical features are related to the compressed structure as follows:

Compression	Clinical Features
Artery	Arm / hand claudication (worse on raising arm above head).
	Acutely ischaemic hand (secondary to emboli).
	Subclavian aneurysm.
Vein	Venous hypertension.
	Arm swelling.
	Venous thrombosis.
Nerve	Motor or sensory deficit (commonly affects the lower 2 nerve roots, C8 & T1).

Special tests for thoracic outlet syndrome include Roo's Test (Fig 7.1) & Adson's Test (Fig 7.2) (*see orthopaedics chapter*).

Q: What are the differential diagnoses for thoracic outlet syndrome?

Classification	Examples
Arterial	Raynaud's Disease / Syndrome
	Thrombangiitis Obliterans
	Takayasu's Arteritis
Venous	Axillary Vein Thrombosis
	Damage to Axillary Drainage e.g. Post-Mastectomy
Neurological	Cervical Spondylosis
	Pancoast Tumour
	Cervical Intervertebral Disc Protrusion
	Ulnar Nerve Neuropathy

Raynaud's Syndrome

Q. What is Raynaud's Syndrome?

This is a syndrome characterised by digital vasospasm, resulting in 3 distinct phases, with visible colour changes noticed in the fingers as follows:

Colour	Cause
White	Arterial spasm causing blanching of the digits (may lead to gangrene).
Blue	Cyanosis & pain caused by insufficient oxygenation.
Red	Reactive hyperaemia once blood flow restored.

Q: How do you classify the causes of Raynaud's Syndrome?

Primary	Secondary
Idiopathic	**Arterial Disorders** e.g. Atherosclerosis
(Raynaud's Disease)	**Blood Disorders** e.g. Polycythaemia
	Connective Tissue Disorders e.g. RA, Scleroderma
	Drugs e.g. β-Blockers, Caffeine, OCP, Smoking
	Trauma e.g. Vibrating Tools (chronic usage)

Q: What is the management of Raynaud's Syndrome?

Conservative	Medical	Surgical
Heated Gloves	Nifedipine	Sympathectomy (commonly thoracoscopic T1-T3, rarely performed open)
Avoid Precipitants e.g. β-Blockers, Caffeine, Cold Weather, OCP, Smoking	α-Blockers	Digital Sympathectomy
	Iloprost Infusion	Amputation (if gangrene present)

Carotid Artery Stenosis

Q: How do you classify carotid artery stenosis?

- Carotid artery stenosis is classified as either **symptomatic** or **asymptomatic**. Symptomatic stenosis is associated with amaurosis fugax, TIA or CVA.

Q. What is the management of carotid artery stenosis?

Conservative	Medical	Surgical
Smoking Cessation	Statins	Carotid Stenting
Exercise	Antihypertensives	Carotid Endarterectomy
Healthy Diet	Aspirin	
	DM control	

Q: What are the indications for carotid endarterectomy?

- Controlled trials have shown that surgery reduces the risk of stroke in symptomatic patients with 50–99% carotid stenosis, more effectively than best medical therapy, if performed within 2 weeks of an event.
- In asymptomatic patients, <75 years, with a significant stenosis, surgery reduces the 5-year risk of stroke by 50%.

Symptomatic patients with >70% stenosis (clear benefit from surgery)
Symptomatic patients with 50–69% stenosis (less benefit from surgery)
Asymptomatic patients with >60% stenosis (some benefit from surgery, especially if male)

Q: How can risk of stroke be estimated after a TIA?

Using the ABCD^2 scoring system:

Risk Factor		Points	2 Day Stroke Risk
Age:	≥60 years	1	Score 0–3 = Low Risk
Blood Pressure:	≥140/90mmHg	1	
Clinical Features:	Unilateral weakness Speech impairment (no weakness)	2 1	Score 4-5 = Moderate Risk
Duration of Symptoms:	≥60mins 10–59mins	2 1	Score 6-7 = High Risk
Diabetes Mellitus:	Present	1	

Deep Vein Thrombosis (DVT)

Q: What is a deep vein thrombosis (DVT)?

Phlebothrombosis of deep veins.

Q: What are the causes of DVT?

Causal factors are related to Virchow's triad, which describes general causes of thrombosis anywhere in the body:

Endothelial Damage	Stasis / Turbulent Blood Flow	Hypercoagulable States
Atheroma	Immobility	Dehydration
Radiotherapy	Obesity	Malignancy
Trauma e.g. Cannulation	Pelvic Surgery	Oral Contraceptive Pill
	Lower Limb Surgery	Hormone Replacement Therapy
	Aneurysm	Smoking
	Cardiac / Vascular Stents	Protein C & S Deficiency
	Cardiac Valve Replacements	Factor V Leiden
	DVT History	Antithrombin Deficiency

Q: What are the clinical features of DVT?

- 75% clinically silent.
- Painful calf / leg swelling that is hot & erythematous.
- Homan's sign = pain on foot dorsiflexion.
- Distended superficial veins due to blockage within deep venous system.
- Phlegmasia alba dolens = painful white leg swelling (iliofemoral vein partial occlusion).
- Phlegmasia caerulea dolens = painful blue leg swelling resulting in gangrene (iliofemoral vein complete occlusion).

Q: What investigations might you consider?

A high index of suspicion is required. Diagnosis involves eliciting risk factors from the history e.g. recent long-haul travel / surgery, thorough examination and confirmation by Duplex scan.

Q: What are the management options?

- Management strategies should be primarily preventative.
- When indicated, treatment-dose low molecular weight heparin (on-ward) may be commenced, with concurrent warfarin treatment until a therapeutic INR is reached.
- The patient may then be discharged on warfarin as per protocol.
- Patients are often anticoagulated for 3 months in the 1st instance.
- With recurrence, anticoagulation may be lifelong.
- Specific treatment strategies include:

Conservative	Mechanical	Medical	Surgical
Maintain Good Hydration	Intermittent Pneumatic Compression Devices	Oral Contraceptive Pill – Stop 4 Weeks Prior to Elective Surgery	Avoid General Anaesthesia if Possible
Leg Exercises		Low Molecular Weight Heparin Prophylaxis	Early Mobilisation After Surgery
Thromboembolic Deterrent Stockings		(IV) Fluids	Vena Cava Filters – Prevent Pulmonary Embolism

Q: What are the complications of DVT?

- The most serious complication is pulmonary embolism & sudden death.
- DVT may also damage venous valves resulting in venous insufficiency & venous hypertensive disease.

Deep Venous Insufficiency & Venous Hypertension

Q: What is deep venous insufficiency?

- Also known as the post-thrombotic / post-phlebitic limb.
- Disruption of the venous return of the deep venous system, with associated valvular incompetence, results in high pressure reflux into superficial veins.

Q: What are the causes?

- Congenital absence of deep vein valves.
- DVT resulting in deep vein valve damage.
- Arterio-venous malformations.

Q: What are the clinical features?

Clinical Features	Notes
Varicose Veins	Tortuous dilated veins, often affecting the lower limbs (see below).
Varicose Eczema	Varicose pruritic rash results in scratching. Potential skin abrasion increases risk of venous ulceration & infection.
Haemosiderin Pigmentation	Venous leak into soft tissues
Lipodermatosclerosis	Silvery-grey patches of skin where fibrous tissue has replaced normal cutaneous tissue.
Peripheral Oedema	May be inflammatory or directly related to venous hypertension & increased intraluminal hydrostatic pressure.
Venous Ulceration	Due to venous hypertension. Scratching results in repeat excoriations. Skin affected by lipodermatosclerosis is less robust, nutrient exchange is decreased & it is therefore more prone to delayed healing. These precipitate a vicious cycle which delays healing.
Infection	Cellulitis most commonly.

Q: What specific investigations would you consider?

- Duplex Scan
- Venography

Q: What are the treatment options?

Treatment is of primarily of the underlying cause & subsequent complications e.g. varicose veins / venous ulceration. Conservative options include avoidance of long periods standing, leg-elevation & compression stockings.

Varicose Veins

Q: What are varicose veins?

- Tortuous dilated veins.
- Most often affecting the long (greater) & short (lesser) saphenous veins of the lower limbs.

Q. What are the causes of varicose veins (Fig 9.3)?

Primary	Secondary
Idiopathic	DVT
Familial	Pregnancy
	Tumour
	Klippel-Trenaunay Syndrome (varicose veins, port-wine stains, soft tissue limb hypertrophy)
	Parkes-Weber Syndrome (AVFs, limb hypertrophy)

Q: What investigations would you consider for varicose veins?

- Diagnosis begins with a full history & thorough clinical examination.
- Investigations must include a venous Duplex scan to assess:
  i. site of incompetence (superficial / deep).
  ii. deep venous system.

Q: What is the management of varicose veins?

After taking a **full history** & performing a **thorough clinical examination**, management should be considered in relation to the underlying cause:

- **Investigations:** Must include a venous Duplex scan to assess (i) the site of incompetence (superficial / deep) & (ii) the deep venous system.
- **Treatment:** May be conservative / surgical *(see below).*

Conservative	Surgical
Support Stockings	Injection Foam Sclerotherapy
Weight Loss & Exercise	Ligation (SFJ / SPJ), Vein Stripping (LSV / SSV) & Stab Avulsions
	Endovenous Laser Therapy (EVLT)
	Radiofrequency Ablation (RFA)

The CLaSS trial (Comparison of Laser, Surgery & Foam Sclerotherapy) is currently underway to identify the most clinical & cost-effective treatment for varicose veins.

Gangrene

Q: What is gangrene?

Gangrene is abnormal & irreversible tissue necrosis due to decreased vascular-nutrient supply (Fig 9.1).

Q: How would you classify gangrene?

Classification	Notes
Dry	Mummification of tissue without infection e.g. peripheral arterial disease.
Wet	Superadded infection, often anaerobic e.g. *Clostridium perfringens / Bacteroides*.
Gas	*Clostridium perfringens* is a gas forming, gram positive anaerobe that produces exotoxin which may cause tissue necrosis, disease spread & local crepitus (palpable crackling of skin due to gas formation).

Q: What are the treatment options for gangrene?

- Treatment strategies are primarily preventative or aimed at the underlying cause.
- Where infection is involved, appropriate antibiotics are used.
- Surgical options include debridement / amputation.

SECTION A4: NEUROSCIENCES

CHAPTER 10
NEUROSCIENCE

V Kakar
BH Miranda
J Nagaria

CHAPTER CONTENTS

Abbreviated Mental Test Score (AMTS)
Mini Mental State Examination (MMS)
Glasgow Coma Scale Assessment (GCS)
Cranial Nerves Examination
Peripheral Nervous System Examination (PNS)
DrExam's Tips for Remembering Myotomes & Nerve Roots
OSCE Questions

- Low Back Pain & Prolapsed Intervertebral Disc
- Cauda Equina Syndrome
- Head Injury *(also see book 1)*
- Traumatic Intracranial Haemorrhage
- Spontaneous Intracranial Haemorrhage
- Stroke (CVA)
- Hydrocephalus
- CNS Infections
- Brain Tumours

ABBREVIATED MENTAL TEST SCORE (AMTS)

This is a screening test consisting of 10 questions.

A score <6/10 suggests dementia / delirium & should precipitate a mini mental state examination.

It is appropriate to perform an AMTS examination on all elderly patients.

Question	Score
How old are you?	1
What is the time (to the nearest hour)?	1
Ask the patient to remember an address e.g. 10 James Street. Explain that you will ask them to recall it at the end of the AMTS examination (do not forget to do this)!	1
What is the year?	1
What is the name of the hospital (or place where the patient is being examined)?	1
Can you identify 2 people (doctor, nurse, family member etc.)?	1
What is your date of birth?	1
What date did World War 2 begin (or another well known date)?	1
Who is the current prime minister (or monarch / president / dictator)?	1
Ask the patient to count backwards from 20 to 1.	1
Total	**10**

MINI MENTAL STATE EXAMINATION (MMS)

This test provides more information than the AMTS with respect to cognitive impairment.

It should be undertaken in all patients who achieve an AMTS score <6/10.

Score 24–30 implies no cognitive impairment.

Score 18–23 implies mild cognitive impairment.

Score 0–17 implies severe cognitive impairment.

Question	Max Score
ORIENTATION	
What is the year? What is the season? What is the date? What month is it? What is the day of the week?	5
What country is this? What region? What city? What hospital is this? What floor?	5
REGISTRATION	
Ask the patient to remember 3 items that you have clearly named e.g. pen, book, shoe. Ask the patient to repeat these items back & record the number of trials it takes for the patient to do this correctly.	3
ATTENTION & CALCULATION	
Ask the patient to count backwards from 100 in 7's until the patent has done this 5 times (93, 86, 79, 72, 65). Alternatively ask the patient to spell WORLD backwards.	5
RECALL	
Can you recall the 3 items that you remembered earlier? (Skip this if the patient was unable to remember the 3 items initially).	3
LANGUAGE & PRAXIS	
Show the patient 2 objects e.g. pen, watch. Ask the patient to name them.	2
Repeat the phrase: *'No ifs, ands or buts.'*	1
Instruct the patient to take a piece of paper in their right hand, fold it in half & put it on the table.	3
Write the following on a piece of paper: *Close your eyes.* Instruct the patient to follow the command that you have written.	1
Instruct the patient to make up any complete sentence & write it on a piece of paper. The sentence must be grammatically accurate.	1
Ask the patient to copy the following picture:	1
Total	**30**

GLASGOW COMA SCALE (GCS)

START: Patient sitting on a chair (unless scenario dictates otherwise).

Ask the patient if they are in pain.

Ask / check for prescription medications that may alter the patient's level of consciousness.

Best Eye Response	Interpretation
4	Open spontaneously
3	Open in response to speech
2	Open in response to pain
1	No response

Best Verbal Response	Interpretation Adults	Interpretation Pre Verbal Children
5	Orientated	Smiles, orientated to sounds, follows objects, interacts
4	Confused	Cries but is consolable, inappropriate interactions
3	Inappropriate speech	Inconsistently consolable, moaning
2	Incomprehensible sounds	Inconsolable, agitated
1	No response	No response

Best Motor Response	Interpretation
6	Obeys commands
5	Localises to pain
4	Flexion withdrawal
3	Abnormal flexion to pain (Decorticate)
2	Abnormal extension to pain (Decerebrate)
1	No response

FINISH:

REMEMBER

- The GCS is a reproducible, objective assessment of a patient's conscious level.
- Assessment in young children can be difficult & a modified verbal scoring system exists.
- GCS ≤8 defines coma & warrants intubation.
- Beware that language barriers may appear to inhibit the patient's response.
- Other trauma may prevent following commands (e.g. spinal injury).

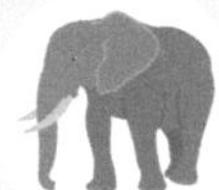

CRANIAL NERVES EXAMINATION

START: Patient sitting on a chair.

Ask the patient if they are in pain.

INSPECTION	Interpretation
Speech	Whilst interacting with the patient at the START of the CNS examination, note any of the following ***3 x D's***: • **Dysarthria:** Disorder of articulation that may be due to alcohol, cerebellar disease, head injury & lesions to cranial nerves V, VII, IX, X, XII. • **Dysphonia:** Disorder of phonation due to vocal organ impairment e.g. vocal cords. • **Dysphasia:** Disorder of language that may be expressive, receptive or mixed
Facial Appearance	Look for ptosis, facial asymmetry & weakness.
Dyskinesia	Look for any movement disorders that may include: • **Fasciculation:** Small involuntary muscular contractions (LMN). • **Tremor:** Involuntary & rhythmical oscillatory muscle movements. • **Dystonia:** Sustained involuntary muscle contractions, resulting in twisting & repetitive movements or abnormal postures. • **Chorea:** Rapid involuntary jerky movements that may be highly variable in location. • **Tic:** Rapid involuntary sudden movements that are stereotypical in location.

CRANIAL NERVES	No.	Interpretation
Olfactory	I	Ask the patient if they have noticed any change in their sense of smell. Test each nostril individually with coffee or chocolate. **Note: Substances e.g. tobacco or ammonia are too noxious & result in trigeminal (V) nerve stimulation.**
Optic	II	Check the following 5 parameters: 1. **Visual Acuity:** Test each eye separately using a **Snellen Chart**. Do this without vision aids, then with best corrected vision e.g. contact lenses, glasses or pinhole camera. Vision is recorded as a fraction, such that normal vision is 6/6. The numerator is the distance that the patient is standing from the chart (metres) & the denominator is the line that the patient can read on the chart. The following should be done in succession until the patient is able to see something, or until no perception of light is detected (in which case NPL should be recorded): • Bring the patient closer to the chart. • Ask the patient how many fingers you are holding up. • Ask the patient to identify your hand movements. • Ask the patient if they can see light. 2. **Visual Fields:** Test each eye separately by confrontation. A red hat pin is best for testing scotomas, as colour vision fails early in optic nerve & retinal disorders. 3. **Colour Vision:** Test each eye separately using **Ishihara Plates**. 4. **Pupils:** Note **size & symmetry**. Test **direct & consensual light reflexes** in a dark room. Test **accommodation**, asking the patient to focus on an object behind you, then on an object close to their face. The normal accommodation reflex for close objects is bilateral pupil constriction. Test **swinging light reflex** for an afferent pathway defect by swinging a pen torch from one eye to the other. Both pupils constrict when the light shines on the normal eye, but when the light shines on the affected eye, that pupil continues to dilate slightly (Marcus Gunn Pupil), indicating optic nerve injury / MS. 5. **Fundoscopy:** Elicit the red reflex & look for any opacities, that will appear dark, outlined by the red glow. Check the optic disc for colour, contour & cupping. Excessive cupping is associated with glaucoma. Assess for indistinct disc margins & lack of retinal venous pulsations (papilloedema). Assess the macula by asking the patient to briefly look straight into the light.
Oculomotor	III	Stabilise the patient's head by gently placing your left hand under the patient's chin. Then, ask the patient to follow your right index finger. Perform the '**H-Manoeuvre**' on each eye separately (Fig 10.1). Remember that eye movements are controlled by III, except for '$\mathbf{SO_{IV}}$' = superior oblique muscle, innervated by IV, adducts the eye with inferior gaze & '$\mathbf{LR_{VI}}$' = lateral rectus, innervated by VI, abducts the eye.
Trochlear	IV	
Abducent	VI	

CHAPTER 10

DrExam™

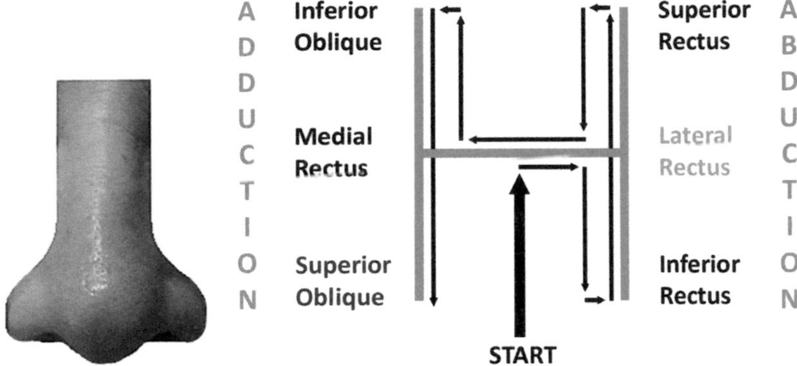

Fig 10.1: The H-Manoeuvre (left eye).

'SO_{IV}' = superior oblique muscle, innervated by IV, adducts the eye with inferior gaze.

'LR_{VI}' = lateral rectus, innervated by VI, abducts the eye.

Note: Arrows represent movement of the pupil.

Trigeminal	**V**	**Sensory:** Assess fine touch, using cotton wool, of the ophthalmic (V1), maxillary (V2) & mandibular (V3) branches (Fig 10.2). Elicit the corneal reflex. **Motor:** Ask the patient to open their mouth. If there is a unilateral lesion affecting the pterygoid muscles, **the jaw will deviate towards the side of the lesion.** **Jaw Jerk:** Put a finger on the patient's mandible, in the midline & gently tap your finger with a tendon hammer. A positive reflex results in masseter activation & jaw closure. This reflex is usually slight or absent. If exaggerated, an UMN lesion is present.
Facial	**VII**	**Facial Asymmetry:** This may have been detected on inspection already. **Sensory:** The chorda tympani nerves may be tested by using a substance that is either salty, sweet, bitter or sour on the anterior ²/₃ of each side of the tongue. **Motor:** Test the branches of the facial nerve by asking the patient to raise their eyebrows, screw up their eyes (against resistance), blow out their cheeks, show their teeth, tense & flare their neck muscles.

Vestibulocochlear	**VIII**	**Hearing:** Ask the patient to reproduce a word that you whisper in their ear. Then perform Rinne's & Weber's Tests as follows: • **Rinne's Test:** Place a vibrating tuning fork (256Hz / 512Hz) on the mastoid process to test bone conduction. When the sound is no longer detected by the patient, place the vibrating arms immediately lateral to the ear. A patient with normal hearing should detect the sound again as air conduction is better than bone conduction. *Conductive hearing loss* may be suspected if the patient is unable to detect the sound again. • **Weber's Test:** Place a vibrating tuning fork on the forehead in the midline. Ask the patient where the sound is heard loudest. A patient with normal hearing should detect the sound equally in the midline. A patient with *conductive hearing loss* will detect the sound loudest in the affected ear. A patient with *sensorineural hearing loss* will detect the sound loudest in the good ear. **Vestibular Function:** Test the oculocephalic reflex in a comatose patient. Slightly flex the neck & quickly rotate the head from side to side. The eyes should move to the left when the patient's head is turned to the right & vice-versa (like doll's eyes).
Glossopharyngeal	**IX**	Test for a gag reflex that may indicate either IX or X pathology. Ask the patient to say 'ahh' & look at the uvula. If there is a unilateral X lesion, **the uvula will deviate away from the side of the lesion**.
Vagus	**X**	
Spinal Accessory	**XI**	Ask the patient to shrug their shoulders against resistance (trapezius). Ask the patient to turn their head to the side against resistance (sternocleidomastoid). *Remember that the sternocleidomastoid laterally rotates the head to the contralateral side.*
Hypoglossal	**XII**	Ask the patient to protrude their tongue. Assess for symmetry, wasting & fasciculations. If there is a unilateral lesion, **the tongue will deviate towards the side of the lesion**.

FINISH:

PERIPHERAL NERVOUS SYSTEM EXAMINATION (PNS)

START: Patient exposed to underwear.

Maintain their dignity.

Chaperone is recommended.

Ensure thorough inspection from the FRONT, BACK & SIDES of the patient.

INSPECTION	Interpretation
Gait	Ask the patient to walk away, turn around & walk back. Comment on any gait abnormalities.
Spine	Comment on abnormal kyphosis, lordosis & scoliosis.
Fasciculation	Look for involuntary muscle contractions.
Wasting	Look for muscle wasting, associated with weakness.
Romberg's Test	Ask the patient to stand with their feet together, arms by their sides & eyes closed. Loss of proprioception will result in loss of stability (positive Romberg's Test).
Cerebellar Signs	Performing a quick cerebellar screen is useful to help fine-tune the candidate's differential diagnosis early on in the examination. A helpful memory aid is **DANISH**: **D**ysdiadochokinesia *(see coordination)* **A**taxia **N**ystagmus **I**ntention Tremor & Past Pointing **S**lurred Speech **H**ypotonia.

Ask about pain.

Ideally, continue with the patient on a couch, lying at 45° (upper limbs) or flat (lower limbs).

Assess tone, power, coordination, sensation & reflexes, remembering to compare each side.

TONE	Interpretation
UPPER LIMB	Hold the patient's hand as if you were going to greet them with a hand shake. Support the patient's upper arm, just proximal to the elbow joint, with your other hand. Tell the patient to relax & 'go floppy' & test tone by quickly moving each joint in succession as follows: • **Shoulder:** Abduction, adduction, flexion, extension, internal & external rotation. • **Ulnar-Humeral Joint:** Flexion & extension of the elbow. • **Radial-Ulnar Joint:** Pronation & supination of the hand / forearm. • **Wrist:** Flexion & extension.

TONE	Interpretation
LOWER LIMB	• Facing the patient's feet, place 1 hand just proximal to each knee joint & quickly roll the knees externally & internally. Look for symmetrical movement of the toes. • Place both hands under the patient's leg, just proximal to the knee & quickly 'flick' each knee off the table. The patient's heel should remain on the examination couch unless there is hypertonia, in which case the heel will also lift off the couch. • Examine for **clonus**, supporting the patient's flexed knee with 1 hand. Quickly dorsiflex the foot & hold this position. Clonus is present if the foot continues to move in a rhythmical manner & is indicative of an UMN lesion.

Muscle movements are tested for power in both the upper & lower limbs.

Remember that the primary goal is to locate particular nerve root pathology.

Ensure that the movements being tested cover the appropriate myotomes.

Compare movements on each side & record the Medical Research Council (MRC) Power Grade *(see box below)*.

POWER	Root	Movement	Muscle	Nerve
UPPER LIMB	**C5**	Shoulder Abduction	Deltoid	Axillary
	C5/C6	Elbow Flexion	Biceps	Musculocutaneous
			Brachioradialis	Radial
	C7/C8	Elbow Extension	Triceps	Radial
	C7	MCPJ Extension	Extensor Digitorum Communis (EDC)	Posterior Interosseous (branch of radial nerve)
	C8	Thumb IPJ Flexion	Flexor Pollicis Longus (FPL)	Anterior Interosseous (branch of median nerve)
	T1	Finger Abduction	Dorsal Interossei	Ulnar
	T1	Thumb Abduction	Abductor Pollicis Brevis (APB)	Median
LOWER LIMB	**L2/L3**	Hip Adduction	Hip Adductors	Obturator
	L2/L3	Hip Flexion	Iliopsoas	Femoral
	L4/L5	Hip Extension	Gluteus Maximus	Sciatic
	L3/L4	Knee Extension	Quadriceps	Femoral
	L5/S1	Knee Flexion	Hamstrings	Sciatic
	L4/L5	Ankle Dorsiflexion	Tibialis Anterior	Deep Peroneal
	S1/S2	Ankle Plantarflexion	Gastrocnemius	Tibial
	L5	Hallux Extension	Extensor Hallucis Longus (EHL)	Deep Peroneal
	L5/S1	Ankle Eversion	Peronei	Superficial Peroneal

UK MRC POWER GRADING:

0: No Movement

1: Contraction Flicker

2: Movement Without Gravity

3: Movement Against Gravity

4: Movement Against Resistance

5: Full Power

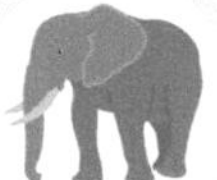

Remember to test both sides for coordination.

COORDINATION	Interpretation
UPPER LIMB	• **Finger–Nose Test:** Place your finger tip within reach of the patient. Ask the patient to touch their nose then your finger tip, each time moving your finger to another position. Then test the contralateral arm. • **Dysdiadochokinesia:** Ask the patient to hold out 1 hand, palmar side up, keeping it still. Instruct the patient to clap this hand with their other hand, rapidly alternating between using the palmar & dorsal surfaces. Then test the contralateral arm. This may have already been tested in the cerebellum screen.
LOWER LIMB	• **Heel–Shin Test:** Ask the patient to use their heel to touch the anterior ankle joint of the contralateral leg. Instruct them to 'sweep' this heel proximally to touch the anterior knee joint, then distally again, **without lifting their heel** off their leg at any time. Then test the contralateral leg.

Remember to test all dermatomes for sensation (Fig 10.2).

SENSATION	Ascending Tract	Interpretation
ANTEROLATERAL SPINOTHALAMIC TRACT	**Pain**	Use a sharp pin & instruct the patient to close their eyes. Test a 'normal' dermatome for 'sharpness'. Instruct the patient to compare this intensity of sharpness quality to the remaining areas being tested. Ask the patient to say 'yes' each time they feel the pin with the same intensity. If they do not respond, ascertain if this intensity is more or less than 'normal'.
	Temperature	Use cold & warm metal tubes, incubated in a beaker of ice & hot water, to test each dermatome. Do this in a similar manner to pain.

SENSATION	Ascending Tract	Interpretation
DORSAL COLUMNS	**Light Touch**	Use a strand of cotton wool to touch each dermatome gently. Do this in a similar manner to pain & do not sweep the strand across the skin.
	Proprioception	Test the position of the DIPJs using gentle extension & flexion. It is important to move the joints by holding the digits on their lateral surfaces, otherwise pressure will guide the patient's interpretation of proprioception. Do this in a similar manner to pain, however the patient should say 'up' or 'down' instead of 'yes'. If proprioception is absent, work proximally until a joint is found where proprioception is preserved. Record this joint.
	2 Point Discrimination	Use a pair of compasses to touch each dermatome. Do this in a similar manner to pain, however the patient should say '1' or '2' points felt instead of 'yes'. Discrimination of 3mm on the pads of the fingers, 1cm on the palm of the hand & 3cm on the sole of the foot is normal.
	Vibration	Use a 128Hz tuning fork to test the dorsal aspects of DIPJs (hand) or IPJ (hallux). Do this in a similar manner to pain. If vibration sensation is absent, move proximally from joint to joint until it is detected.

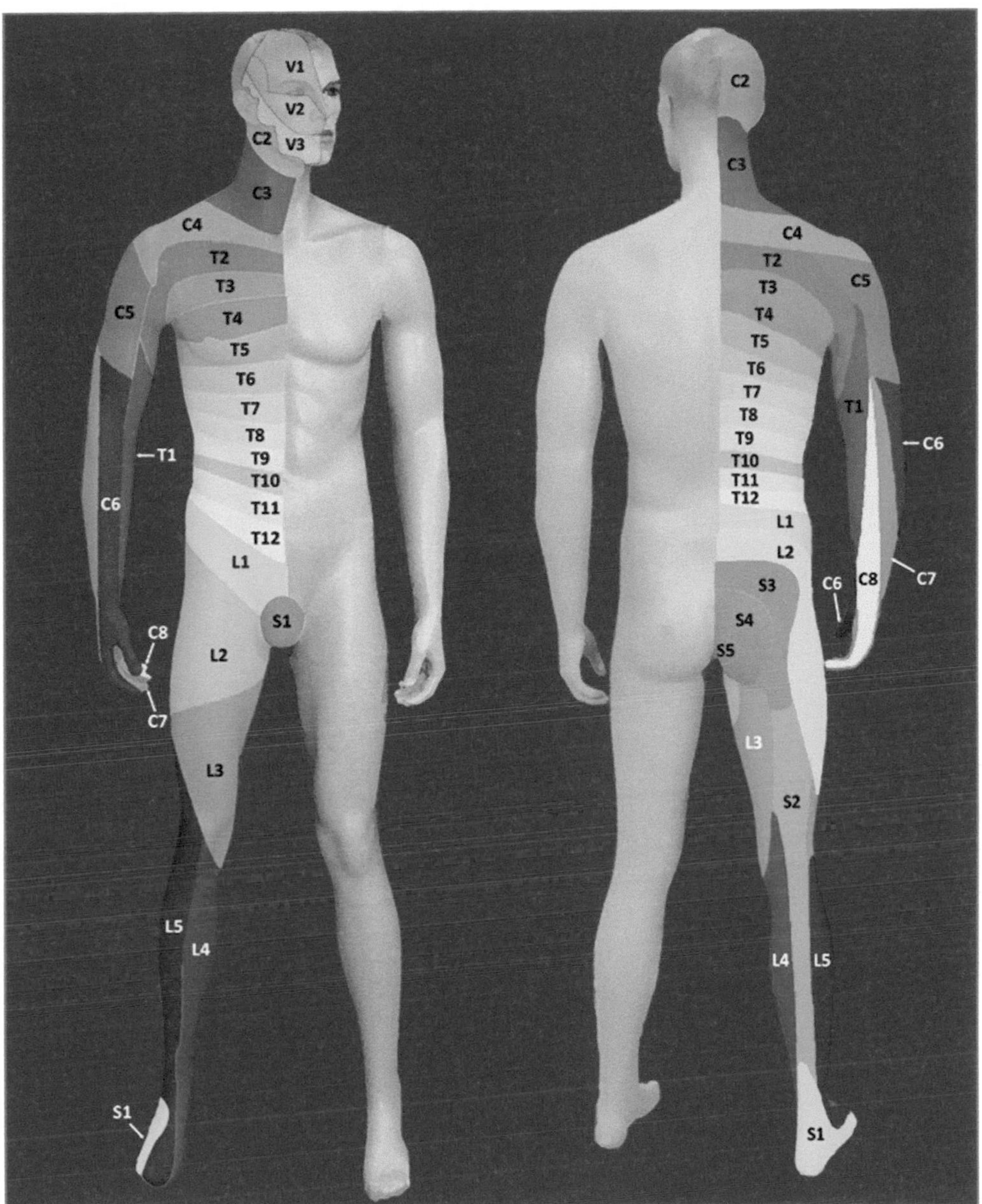

Fig 10.2: Dermatomes of the body. Left = anterior view. Right = posterior view.

CHAPTER 10

NEUROSCIENCE EXAMINATION

Remember to test both sides for reflexes on both sides & compare each side.

Grade the reflex response where possible *(see box below).*

REFLEXES	Arc	Interpretation
Ankle	**S1/S2**	Abduct & externally rotate the patient's hip & flex their knee. Use your hand to slightly plantarflex the foot at the ankle. Using the tendon hammer, strike the patient's Achilles tendon swiftly & accurately. The foot should be seen to plantarflex in response.
Knee	**L3/L4**	Support the patient's leg by 'hooking' your arm underneath, just proximal to the knee. Position the leg, flexed at the hip, so that the knee is flexed to approximately 60°. Using the tendon hammer, strike the patient's infrapatellar tendon swiftly & accurately. The knee should be seen to extend in response.
Biceps	**C5/C6**	Position the patient's arm, adducted at the shoulder & slightly flexed at the elbow, resting across their body. Place the pulp of your thumb on the biceps tendon. Using the tendon hammer, strike your thumb swiftly & accurately using a pendular motion. The biceps tendon should contract in response. This will be felt under the pulp of the thumb.
Supinator	**C5/C6**	Position the patient's arm as for the biceps reflex, ensuring the arm is slightly pronated. Place your index & middle fingers on the radial border of the patient's radius, approximately 5cm proximal to the wrist. Using the tendon hammer, strike your fingers swiftly & accurately. The elbow should be seen to flex, accompanied by finger flexion. If finger flexion only is observed, a spinal cord lesion involving C5 or C6 may be present. This response is termed an inverted reflex & may be associated with an absent biceps jerk. Causes of an inverted reflex include trauma, syringomyelia & prolapsed intervertebral disc.
Triceps	**C7/C8**	Position the patient's arm as for the biceps reflex & lean on the patient's resting hand. Using the tendon hammer, strike the patient's triceps tendon swiftly & accurately. The triceps muscle should be seen to contract in response.
Babinski	**L4–S2**	Immobilise the patient's leg by placing a firm hand just proximal to the ankle joint. Using the tendon hammer tip, purposefully swipe the lateral aspect of the foot in a proximal-distal motion. Whilst you are doing this, look at the toes for a flicker of motion that usually occurs as the tip reaches the level of the ball of the foot. The moment this flicker is detected, swipe the tip across the ball of the foot in a lateral-medial motion. The toes should be seen to flex. If an UMN lesion is present, the toes will abduct & extend.
Abdominal	**T7–T12**	Ensure the patient is lying completely relaxed. Use the tendon hammer tip to gently stroke the periumbilical skin, anticlockwise in a continuous motion. Each quadrant of the abdomen should be seen to contract as the tip enters the region.
Cremasteric	**L1/L2**	Gently stroke the proximal-medial aspect of the thigh. The ipsilateral testicle should be seen to retract.

REFLEXES	Arc	Interpretation
Anal	**S2–S4**	Prick the skin at the anal margin. The anal sphincter should be seen to contract. This is important in suspected cauda equina syndrome as it may often be absent. **Memory: S2/S3/S4 keeps the faeces off the floor!**
Bulbocavernosus	**S2–S4**	Squeeze the glans penis, clitoris or tug on an indwelling urinary catheter. The anal sphincter should be felt to contract. After spinal trauma, presence of this reflex with no motor / sensory function implies complete injury & suggests poor prognosis.

GRADING REFLEXES:

0	Absent
±	Present With Reinforcement
+	Hyporeflexia
++	Normal
+++	Hyperreflexia
++++	Hyperreflexia & Clonus

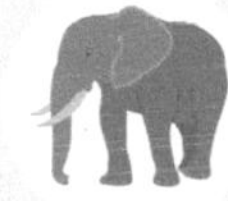

FINISH:

DrEXAM'S TIPS FOR REMEMBERING MYOTOMES & NERVE ROOTS

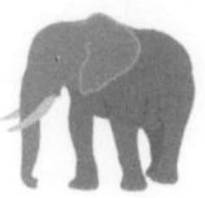

Myotomes & dermatomes are often feared by OSCE candidates, however there is no need to be afraid! A number of recognisable patterns exist & this knowledge may be 'layered' as follows:

1. Learn the arcs for the main limb reflexes first:

Memory:	**1,2,3,4,5,6,7,8**
Ankle:	S1/S2
Knee:	L3/L4
Biceps:	C5/C6
Triceps:	C7/C8

2. Note that the **myotomes correspond to the reflex arcs** i.e. ankle plantarflexion = S1/S2, knee extension = L3/L4, elbow flexion = C5/C6 & elbow extension = C7/C8. You now know 2 major myotomes for both the upper & lower limbs, so it should now be easier to work out the remaining myotomes!
3. Note some **important patterns in the lower limb** as follows:

Anterior movements of the lower limb begin with the last nerve root from the proximal joint, hence hip flexion = L2/L3, knee extension = L3/L4, ankle dorsiflexion = L4/L5.

Posterior movements of the lower limb begin with the last nerve root from the proximal joint, hence hip extension = L4/L5, knee flexion = L5/S1, ankle plantarflexion = S1/S2.

Anterior & posterior movements of the same joint follow directly on from each other, hence hip flexion & extension = L2/L3 & L4/L5, knee extension & flexion = L3/L4 & L5/S1, ankle dorsiflexion & plantarflexion = L4/L5 & S1/S2.

4. **Practise these movements** on your own limbs. This also applies for the dermatomes.

OSCE QUESTIONS

Low Back Pain & Prolapsed Intervertebral Disc

Q: What is the epidemiology of low back pain?

- Lifetime incidence >85%.
- It is the most common reason for disability in patients aged <45 years.
- No significant sex / race differences.
- Prevalence increases with age & pregnancy.

Q: What are the causes of low back pain?

Classification	Examples
Congenital	Kyphosis, Scoliosis, Spina Bifida, Spondylolisthesis.
Degenerative	OA, Spondylosis, Facet Joint Hypertrophy.
Gynaecological	Endometriosis, Pelvic Inflammatory Disease, Tumours.
Infective	Osteomyelitis , TB, Discitis.
Inflammatory	Ankylosing Spondylitis.
Metabolic	Osteoporosis.
Musculoskeletal	Posture Related Muscle Spasm (commonly in the lumbar region).
Neurological	Spinal Canal Stenosis, Prolapsed Intervertebral Disc, Spinal Haematoma.
Neoplastic	Primary (uncommon), Secondary Metastases (more common).
Psychiatric	Functional Overlay.
Renal	Calculi, Renal Cell Carcinoma.
Traumatic	Vertebral Fractures, Muscle Tears, Ligamentous Injuries.
Vascular	AAA.

Q: What is the mechanism of a prolapsed intervertebral disc?

- Posterior herniation of the central nucleus pulposus, through the annulus fibrosis, into the spinal canal.
- 50% are at the level L4/5 & 40% at L5/S1.
- Caused by a degenerative cascade, described in stages as follows:

Stage	Mechanism	Clinical Features
Dysfunction	'Acute' injury. Tear of the annulus fibrosis & prolapse of the inner nucleus pulposus with cartilage destruction. An inflammatory facet joint reaction occurs.	Back pain (worse on movement), localised tenderness on palpation, muscle spasm. Significant prolapse may impinge nerve root(s) causing radiculopathy or cauda equina syndrome.
Instability	Disc resorption & loss of height. Facet joints may become lax, predisposing to subluxation.	Intermittent back pain. Possible detectable instability on movement. Neurological deficit may persist or worsen.
Restabilisation	Osteophyte formation & progressive stenosis.	Chronic back pain but with reduced severity. Neurological deficits stabilise.

Q: What investigations would help your diagnosis of a prolapsed intervertebral disc?

After taking a full history & performing a thorough clinical examination, I would consider the following diagnostic investigations:

Investigation	Notes
MRI (gold standard)	Urgent if cauda equina syndrome is suspected *(see below)* (Fig 10.3).
CT (myelogram)	In absence of MRI / MRI contraindicated.

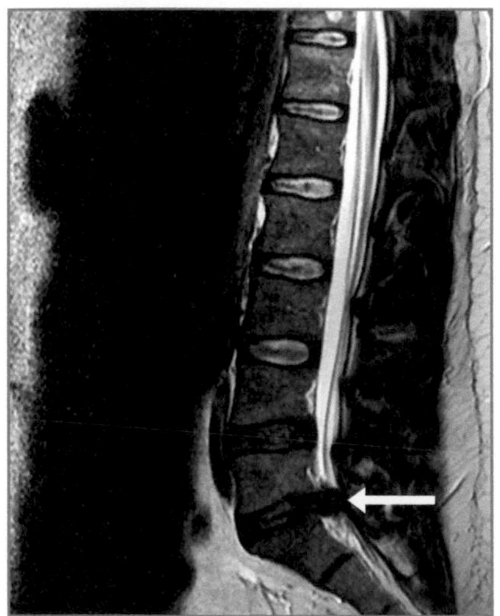

Fig 10.3: Sagittal T2 weighted lumbar spine MRI demonstrating a large disc prolapsed at the L5 / S1 level.

Q: What are the clinical features of lumbar radiculopathy secondary to a prolapsed intervertebral disc?

These are dependent on the level of involvement as follows:

L4 / L5 (compression of ipsilateral L5 nerve root)	L5 / S1 (compression of ipsilateral S1 nerve root)
L5 dermatome pain & sensory impairment	S1 dermatome pain & sensory impairment
Weak foot dorsiflexion	Weak foot plantarflexion
Weak extensor hallucis longus	Depressed / absent ankle jerk

Q: What are the treatment options for lumbar radiculopathy, secondary to a prolapsed intervertebral disc?

Conservative	Medical	Surgical
Lifestyle Modification & Patient Education	Analgesic Ladder	Lumbar Discectomy (>90% improvement, 5% recurrence rate)
OT / PT	Epidural & Nerve Root Injections	Lumbar Discectomy & Laminectomy (for canal stenosis)
Heat / Hydrotherapy		Lumbar Arthrodesis (for spondylosis)
TENS Machine		

Note: <20% of patients will require surgical intervention. Indications for surgery include cauda equina syndrome, intractable pain & progressive motor deficit (MRC Grade ≤3).

Cauda Equina Syndrome

Q: What is cauda equina syndrome & what are the characteristic features?

Cauda equina syndrome results from compression of the cauda equina nerve roots, secondary to a prolapsed intervertebral disc (most commonly) & constitutes a surgical emergency. Other causes include haematoma, infection, inflammatory conditions, malignancy & trauma.

Q: What are the clinical features of cauda equina syndrome?

Clinical features are characterised by the following 'red flags':

- Severe Low Back Pain
- Bilateral Sciatica
- Saddle Anaesthesia & Genital Sensory Deficit
- Bowel & Bladder Sphincter Dysfunction
- Sexual Dysfunction

3 typical presentations are well recognised:

1. **Sudden Onset** (in previously 'well' patient)
2. **Acute Bladder / Bowel Dysfunction** (in patient with low back pain & sciatica)
3. **Gradual Progression** (no acute / rapid deterioration)

Q: How would you classify cauda equina syndrome?

This may be classified as incomplete or complete as follows:

Incomplete	Complete
Difficulty urinating	Painless urinary retention ± overflow
Altered sensation on defecating	Altered / no sensation on defecating
Unilateral / partial perianal & genital sensory deficit	Bilateral perianal & genital sensory deficit
Some residual anal tone	Absent anal tone

Q: What questions are important to ask in the history & what examination features are essential to document in cauda equina syndrome?

When taking a full history & performing a thorough examination, I would ensure that the following are addressed:

History	Examination
Do you have pain in both legs? Is it worse than the back pain?	Assess & document genital sensation.
When did you last pass urine / open your bowels?	Assess & document perianal sensation & anal sphincter tone (per rectum examination).
Do you have difficulty urinating? Is there dribbling / leakage?	On catheterisation, document residual urine & catheter tug sensation.
Can you feel the paper when you wipe your bottom?	Document lower limb tone, power, coordination, sensation & reflexes.
Do you have numbness in your bottom & genitals?	

Q: What are the treatment options for cauda equina syndrome caused by disc prolapse?

This is a neurosurgical emergency as irreversible nerve ischaemia begins to occur at 6 hours. Surgical decompression is via discectomy & decompressive laminectomy of 1–2 vertebrae typically. Incomplete cauda equina syndrome has a good prognosis if surgery is performed <12 hours of onset. Complete cauda equina syndrome has a limited prognosis, however reasonable recovery may still occur if surgery is performed <24 hours of onset.

Head Injury

(also see book 1 critical care chapter)

Q What is the epidemiology of head injuries?

- Estimated 1,000,000 A&E attendances per year.
- Approximately 200,000 hospital admissions.
- Approximately 4,000 patients undergo neurosurgery for head injury per year.

Q: What important specific points would you consider in the history of a patient with a suspected head injury?

History	Notes	
Mechanism	Was there a history of assault, falls or RTA? If there is a history of falls, ascertain any precipitating syncopal events.	
Loss of Consciousness	What was the duration? Was it witnessed? Obtain 3rd-party history if possible.	
Amnesia	**Retrograde:**	Unable to recall events prior to the injury.
	Anterograde:	Unable to recall events after the injury.
Raised ICP Symptoms	Headache, nausea & vomiting, visual disturbances, focal neurological deficit.	
General	Medical & surgical co-morbidities, medications e.g. anticoagulants / antiplatelets, allergies, last meal.	

Q: What signs would you look for to confirm a head injury?

Specific points to consider include:

Examination	Notes
External Trauma	Ecchymoses, lacerations, haemorrhage.
Base of Skull Fracture	Periorbital bruising (**panda / raccoon eyes**), retroauricular bruising (**Battle's Sign**), CSF otorrhoea / rhinorrhoea, bleeding from ear / behind tympanic membrane.
GCS	Compare at scene & post-resuscitation. GCS ≤8 is associated with a need for intubation.
Pupils	Asymmetry, reaction to light.
Focal Neurological Deficit	Cranial nerve palsy, limb motor weakness, sensory deficit.
Associated Spinal Trauma	Bruising, vertebral fractures, poor anal sphincter tone (PR).

Q: When would you request a CT brain (& cervical spine) after a head injury?

These are based on NICE guidelines & include:

CT Modality	Notes
Immediate CT Brain	**Absolute Indications:** • GCS <13 on initial assessment in A&E • GCS <15 more than 2 hours after injury • Suspected open, depressed or base of skull fracture • Post traumatic seizure • Focal neurological deficit • ≥2 or episodes of vomiting (≥3 in children) • Amnesia of events >30 minutes before impact **Consider High Risk Criteria:** • Age >65 years • Coagulopathy • Dangerous mechanism of injury e.g. ejection from vehicle, pedestrian vs vehicle
CT Cervical Spine (in addition to brain)	• GCS <13 on initial assessment in A&E • Intubated patient • Suspected abnormality on plain film or technically inadequate • Patient being scanned for multi-region trauma

Q: How would you classify the severity of a head injury?

According to whether it is **open** (stabbing, gunshot, compound fracture) or **closed** (blunt trauma) & according to GCS as follows:

Minor (80%)	Moderate (10%)	Severe (10%)
GCS 14–15	GCS 9–13	GCS ≤8

Q: When would you refer a patient with a head injury to a neurosurgeon?

All moderate & severe head injuries should be discussed with a neurosurgeon. In addition, the following criteria necessitate discussion:

- New 'surgically significant' abnormality on CT
- GCS ≤8 persisting after resuscitation
- Unexplained confusion >4 hours
- Deterioration in GCS (by ≥2 points)
- Progressive focal neurological deficit
- Seizure without full recovery
- Open or suspected open injury
- CSF leak

Q: What are the principles of management of a minor head injury in a non-neuroscience centre?

- Manage according to ATLS resuscitation principles.
- For patients admitted with GCS = 15, observations should include RR, pulse, BP, saturations, GCS, pupils & focal neurological deficit & should be:

  ½ hourly for first 2 hours
  Hourly for next 4 hours
  2 hourly thereafter.
- Ensure adequate analgesia (caution with opiates).
- Ensure adequate hydration & check electrolytes (especially Na^+).
- Consider antiepileptics (discuss with neurosurgeon).
- Consider rescan & rediscussion with neurosurgeon if GCS deteriorates, worsening headache, nausea or vomiting.
- Consider referral to neurorehabilitation for post concussional syndrome.

Q: What are the indications for emergency neurosurgery following head injury?

Depends on individual circumstances (age, neurological status, co-morbidities, other injuries) but the following are a guide:

- Extradural or subdural haematoma with >5mm midline shift.
- Intracerebral haematoma >40cm^3 in surgically accessible area.
- Depressed skull fracture with depression > skull thickness.
- Potentially all open injuries for wound exploration *(no role for prophylactic antibiotics in base of skull fractures).*

Q: What are the management principles for severe head injuries that *do not* require immediate neurosurgery?

Primary Goals:

Prevention of secondary brain injury, cerebral ischaemia & herniation. A rise in ICP generally results in a fall in CPP, with a reduction in O_2 supply (resulting in ischaemia) & CO_2 clearance (resulting in vasodilation). This precipitates a vicious cycle that worsens brain injury & increases ICP further.

General Management Principles:

- Follow ATLS principles for patients with multi-system trauma.
- Intubation & ventilation in ICU.
- Insertion of ICP monitor (see ICP section).

*Aim is to optimise potential for recovery using medical & surgical strategies to maintain:

- CPP > 65 mmHg
- ICP < 25 mmHg

Specific Management Principles:

The following specific measures are considered in a stepwise 'tiered' fashion depending on response:

Tier	Medical	Surgical
1	• **Elevate Head (30–45°).** • ***Avoid Hypoxia & Hypercapnoea.*** • **Sedation & Paralysis:** Decreases O_2 demand & cerebral blood flow, therefore decreasing ICP. • **Control P_aCO_2 (4-4.5kPa):** Moderate hyperventilation 'blows off' CO_2 to help prevent cerebral vasodilation. • **Maintain MAP:** This helps maintain CPP. • **Ensure Normothermia.**	• **External Ventricular Drainage.** Therapeutic CSF withdrawal to control ICP.
2	*Tier 1 +* • **Increase Sedation**: Use boluses if required. • **Induce Hypothermia (33-35°C):** Reduces metabolic demand. • **Mannitol** (osmotic diuretic) / **Hypertonic Saline** (target Na^{2+} 145-155mmol/l)**:** Reduces cerebral oedema. There is a risk of renal impairment when serum osmolality >320mOsm/kg water.	• **External Ventricular Drainage**: Therapeutic CSF withdrawal to control ICP.
3	*Tiers 1 & 2 +* • **Barbiturate Coma** (e.g. thiopentone)**:** Induces 'total cerebral narcosis' & reduces brain metabolic demand to minimum requirement. Risks include myocardial depression, hepatic & renal impairment.	*Tiers 1 & 2 +* • **Consider Decompressive Craniectomy:** Remove skull section(s) to allow cerebral herniation into defect.

Q: What are the possible neurological sequelae for survivors of severe head injury?

Sequela	Notes
Vegetative State	No Physical Recovery
Cognitive Impairment	Concentration & Memory Impairment
Epilepsy	Partial / General Seizures
Location Specific	**Brainstem:** 'Locked In' Syndrome **Frontal:** Disinhibition, Emotional Disturbance, Personality Disorder **Temporal:** Aphasia **Motor Cortex:** Mono-, Hemi- or Tetraparesis
Psychiatric	Delirium, Depression, Psychosis

Traumatic Intracranial Haemorrhage

Q: What are the most common causes of intracranial heamorrhage?

1. Trauma (most common)
2. Spontaneous Intracerebral Heamorrhage (heamorrhagic stroke)
3. Subarchnoid Haemorrhage

Q: What are the underlying mechanisms & features of traumatic intracranial haemorrhages?

Classification & Location		Mechanism & Features
EXTRA-AXIAL	**Extradural Haematoma (EDH) (Fig 10.4)**	• High pressure arterial origin (middle meningeal artery most commonly). • >85% associated with skull fracture. • Decreased GCS & contralateral hemiparesis is common. • <30% have classic presentation of LOC → lucid interval → rapid deterioration ('talk & die'). • Variable underlying brain injury is present. • High density bi-convex lesion on non-contrast CT scan.
	Subdural Haematoma (SDH) (Fig 10.5)	• Generally venous origin. • Cortical laceration in young (often with significant underlying brain injury). • Bridging veins between inner table of skull & brain in elderly. • Decreased GCS & contralateral hemiparesis is common. • High density, concave lesion on non contrast CT scan.
INTRA-AXIAL	**Intracerebral Haematoma / Contusion (ICH) (Fig 10.6)**	• Due to direct brain injury. • Most commonly in inferior frontal lobe & temporal lobe due to anatomy of skull base (85%). • Decreased GCS & focal neurological deficit is characteristic. • Symptoms may worsen after 24–48 hours. • High density lesion in affected area on CT scan, with surrounding low density (cytotoxic) oedema. • **Coup** = direct injury. • **Contrecoup** = injury on opposite side of direct injury.

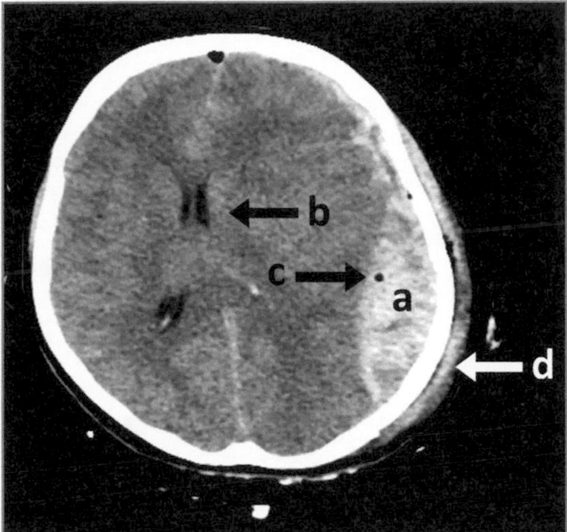

Fig 10.4: Axial CT brain (non contrast) demonstrating large left parietal / frontal extradural haematoma (EDH) (a) with midline shift (b). There are locules of air (c) within the EDH that may suggest an actively enlarging haematoma or possible open injury. There is also an extracranial scalp haematoma (d).

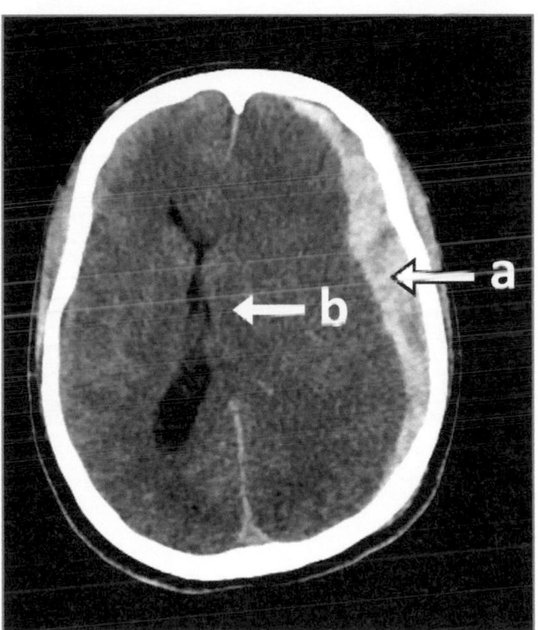

Fig 10.5: Axial CT brain (non contrast) demonstrating large left acute subdural haematoma (SDH) (a) & midline shift (b).

Q: What are the management options for traumatic intracranial haemorrhages?

Management is according to ATLS resuscitation & head injury principles *(see head injuries)*. Specific options include:

Extradural	Subdural	Intracerebral
Conservative (if small)	**Conservative** (if small / chronic)	**Conservative** (mostly)
Endovascular Embolisation (if small & stable)	**Consider Trial of Steroids** (if chronic)	**Craniotomy & Evacuation** (if >40cm^3 or with inferior temporal lobe / cerebellum involvement due to risk of brainstem compression)
Craniotomy & Evacuation (if increasing in size / >0.5cm thick with >5mm midline shift / deteriorating GCS)	**Burr Hole Drainage** (if chronic with mass effect)	**Bifrontal Decompressive Craniectomy** (consider for small, diffuse bifrontal contusions with mass effect)
	Craniotomy & Evacuation (if >1cm thick with midline shift / focal neurological deficit / deteriorating GCS)	**Note: Delayed deterioration is common due to 'maturation' of contusions, peaking at days 3–6.**

Spontaneous Intracranial Haemorrhage

Q: What is the difference between intracerebral & subarachnoid haemorrhage?

Haemorrhage	Notes
Intracerebral	Haemorrhage into brain parenchyma (Intra-axial)
Subarachnoid	Haemorrhage into subarachnoid space (Extra-axial)

Q: What are the risk factors for spontaneous intracerebral haemorrhage?

Spontaneous intracerebral haemorrhage has an annual incidence of approximately 10–15 / 100,000. >80% are secondary to hypertension & amyloidosis. Risk factors include:

Classification	Examples
Unavoidable	• **Age** (>55 years) • Race (Afro-Caribbean > Caucasian)
Iatrogenic	• Post Operative (especially malignant tumours)
Medical	• Coagulopathy (hepatic failure / antigcoagulation) • **Hypertension (affects basal ganglia & brainstem)** • **Amyloidosis (amyloid angiopathy weakens blood vessel walls)**
Vascular	• Aneurysm • AVM
Social	Illicit Drugs The most common cause in patients <30 years (amphetamines, cocaine)

Q: What are the treatment principles of spontaneous intracerebral haemorrhage?

Conservative	Medical	Surgical
Modify Risk Factors	Resuscitation	Craniotomy & Evacuation
	Control Hypertension	
	Reverse Anticoagulation	

Note: Current evidence base overall does not support surgical intervention. In general, right hemisphere peripheral parietal haematomas are most favourable for surgery. Basal ganglia & brainstem haematomas are least favourable for surgery.

Q: What is the epidemiology of subarachnoid haemorrhage?

- Annual incidence 10–15 per 100,000 (not changed in last 40 years)
- Increased prevalence in patients aged 50–65 years
- Sex difference (female : male = 1.5 : 1)
- Race difference (Afro-Caribbean : Caucasian = 2 : 1)

Note: Estimated prevalence of intracranial aneurysms is 4-7%. This implies that that most aneurysms *do not* rupture & remain asymptomatic.

Q: What are the causes of subarachnoid haemorrhage?

Approximately 80% are due to rupture of an aneurysm. 15% of patients have multiple aneurysms. Causes may therefore be classified as follows:

Cause	Notes
Idiopathic	No cause found
Aneurysm	Berry Aneurysm (saccular) Rupture >75% Infective e.g. Endocarditis Inflammatory
Arteriovenous Malformation	AVM Dural Arteriovenous Fistula (these are mostly acquired)
Trauma	Uncommon & usually with a different radiological distribution of blood vs. spontaneous bleeds.

Q: What features on history & examination suggest subarachnoid haemorrhage?

Consider in any patient presenting with a sudden onset, severe headache. 5–10% die immediately & 15% are comatose on arrival to A&E. Also consider the following headache history & examination findings:

Headache History	Examination
Very Sudden Onset (reaching maximum intensity <1min)	**May Be Entirely Normal**
Persisting	**Meningism**
Usually Worst Ever Experienced	**Focal Neurological Deficit** (hemiparesis / monoparesis) (cranial nerve (III) palsy = posterior communicating artery aneurysm)
Variable Location (classically occipital)	**Visual Defect** (ophthalmic artery aneurysm)
Dull / Boring Character	**Papilloedema** (uncommon acutely as develops >6 hours from onset)
Associated Nausea & Vomiting	**Drowsiness**
Associated LOC	**Coma**
Associated Seizure	

Q: What investigations would you order / perform to confirm subarachnoid haemorrhage?

Investigation	Examples
CT Brain (Fig 10.6) (non-contrast)	• Sensitivity >96% in 1st 6 hours. • Sensitivity drops to 80% at 3 days. • CT is generally superior to MRI for detecting SAH.
Lumbar Puncture	• If CT is normal, perform at >12hours. • Sensitivity drops with time but is still worth doing up to 14 days. • CSF bilirubin indicates SAH. • A raised oxyhaemoglobin level may cause a false negative bilirubin reading. • Must obtain CSF WCC, RBC count, protein, oxyhaemoglobin & bilirubin absorbance ratios.

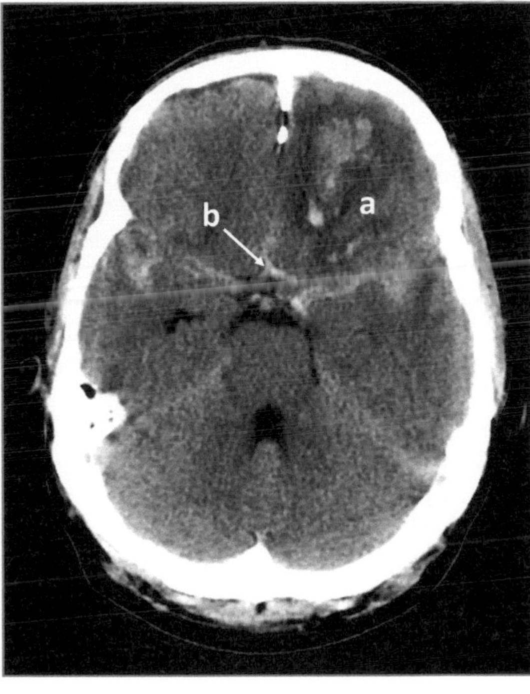

Fig 10.6: Axial CT brain (non contrast) at the level of the Circle of Willis. There is patchy intracerebral haemorrhage (ICH) in the left frontal lobe (a) & diffuse subarachnoid haemorrhage (SAH) in the basal cisterns (b).

Q: What radiological investigations would you order to detect an intracranial aneurysm?

- **CT- Angiogram** (detects most aneurysms, except the smallest)
- **MR- Angiogram** (better detection at skull base than CT)
- **Catheter Angiogram** ('gold standard' but invasive & carries 1/1000 risk of stroke)

Q: What are the treatment options for a proven aneurysmal subarachnoid haemorrhage?

Treatment is aimed at securing the aneurysm & reducing the risk of re-bleeding:

Treatment	Notes
Conservative	Supportive treatment should be considered in patients with a poor recovery from an initial SAH, elderly patients & patients with major co-morbidities.
Interventional	Endovascular embolisation with coils (for >80% of patients with aneurysms in the UK, but only 50% in USA). Procedure involves femoral catheterisation, passage of microcatheter**s** to the cerebral vasculature & deployment of coils into the aneurysm sac. This is most suitable for aneurysms with a large dome & narrow neck. Some require stent assistance to assist access.
Surgical	Craniotomy & titanium clipping of the aneurysm neck (prevents aneurysm filling). Performed when coiling has failed, is technically unfeasible or when there is an existing requirement for craniotomy e.g. evacuation of large haematoma due to SAH.

Stroke (CVA)

Q: What is a stroke?

Clinical syndrome, with an underlying vascular cause, of rapidly developing clinical features of focal or global disturbance in cerebral function lasting >24h or leading to death.

*Note: Transient ischaemic attacks (TIAs) are similar, however clinical features last <24h.

Q: What is the epidemiology?

- 3rd most common cause of death in developed countries.
- Affects 200 per 100000 people per year.
- Commonly in 65-75 year age group.
- Significant cause of morbidity in aging populations

Q: What is the pathophysiology of stroke?

- Cerebrovascular accidents (CVAs / strokes) may be **haemorrhagic** *(see spontaneous Intracranial haemorrhage section),* **thrombotic** or **embolic**.
- Thrombotic CVAs are due to atherosclerosis resulting in atheroma formation within the affected blood vessel and subsequent acute occlusion.
- Embolic CVAs most commonly originate from a site of thrombus e.g. at the carotid artery bifurcation / from the cardiac atria in AF. Other emboli include fat, air & foreign bodies.
- The result of the above CVA mechanisms is brain parenchyma damage (Fig 10.7).

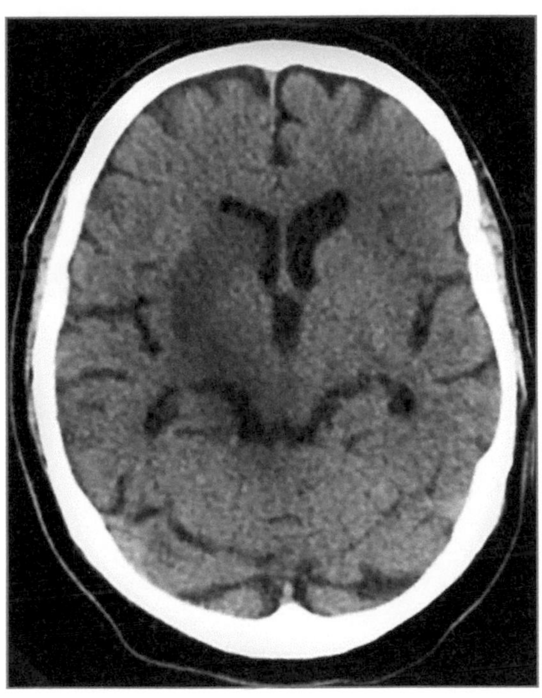

Fig 10.7: Embolic CVA CT.

CT scan illustrating right middle cerebral artery infarction.

Q: What are the risk factors for stroke?

These may be classified as non-modifiable & modifiable as follows:

Non-Modifiable	Modifiable
Age	Hypertension
Gender (more common in males)	Hypercholesterolaemia
Diabetes	Obesity
Genetic Predisposition	Poor Diet
Essential Medications e.g. Warfarin (haemorrhagic stroke)	Smoking
	Alcohol
	Sedentary Lifestyle
	Stress

Q: What are the management strategies for stroke?

- Hospital admission for thorough investigation & diagnosis (CT / Angiogram).
- Treatment:

Preventative measures are most important, medical & surgical treatment options depend on the underlying pathology e.g. anticoagulants & thrombolysis are contraindicated in haemorrhagic strokes. Treatment options include:

Prevention	Medical	Surgical
Reduce Risk Factors	Anticoagulants	Carotid Endarterectomy
Treat Predisposing Conditions	Thrombolysis	Superficial Temporal to Middle Cerebral Artery Anastomosis
	Calcium Antagonists e.g. Nimodipine	
	Aspirin	
	Good INR Control (if on warfarin)	

- Risk factor identification & reduction e.g. on a stroke unit.
- Rehabilitation e.g. physiotherapy & occupational therapy.
- Care plan implementation e.g. district nurse / care home.
- Psychological support.

Hydrocephalus

Q: What is hydrocephalus?

- Hydrocephalus is an imbalance between CSF production & absorption usually due to increased CSF volume & pressure.
- May cause increased ICP, progressive head enlargement, convulsions, mental disability, coma & death.

Q: What do you know about CSF production?

- Average adult ventricular system contains 150mls CSF.
- CSF is produced by the **choroid plexus** & **ependyma** at 20mls/hour (480mls/day).
- CSF is reabsorbed by the **arachnoid villi**.

 How would you classify hydrocephalus?

Classification	Sub-Classification	Examples
INCREASED CSF PRODUCTION	(rare)	• Choroid Plexus Papilloma. • Choroid Plexus Carcinoma.
IMPAIRED CSF CIRCULATION	**Obstructive:** Impairment within ventricular system. Ventricles DO NOT communicate with subarachnoid space.	• Congenital Aqueduct Stenosis (obstructs aqueduct of Sylvius). • Congenital Arnold-Chiari Malformation (obstruction at foramen magnum). • Thalamic Tumour (obstructs 3rd ventricle). • Cerebellar Tumour (obstructs 4th ventricle).
	Communicating: Impairment within subarachnoid space. Ventricles DO communicate with subarachnoid space.	• Head Injury. • Infection e.g. brain abscess / meningitis. • Subarachnoid Haemorrhage.
IMPAIRED CSF ABSORPTION	–	• Sinus Thrombosis. • Subarachnoid Haemorrhage. • Superior Vena Cava Syndrome.
Other	–	• Benign Intracranial Hypertension. • Normal Pressure Hydrocephalus.

Q: How does hydrocephalus present?

This depends on several factors including patient age, speed & duration of onset & cause. Clinical features may generally be classified according to onset as follows:

Classification	Examples
Acute (hours – days)	• **Infants:** Poor feeding, drowsiness / irritability, bulging anterior fontanelle, 'sunsetting' eyes (downward gaze & lid retraction = Parinaud's Syndrome), distended scalp veins, increasing head circumference. • **Adults:** Severe headache, nausea & vomiting, visual disturbance, gait disturbance, focal neurological deficit, papilloedema, drowsiness, coma.
Subacute (days – weeks)	More insidious onset with morning headaches, nausea & vomiting, upward gaze failure, delayed deterioration after an initial recovery.
Chronic (months)	Cognitive impairment, gait disturbance, bowel incontinence, neck pain.

Q: What imaging would you request for hydrocephalus?

After taking a **full history** & performing a **thorough clinical examination**, I would consider the following:

Imaging	Notes
USS	Useful for infants & may be done on ward (via anterior fontanelle).
CT	Reveals ventricular size & configuration.
MRI	Reveals small space occupying lesions missed on CT & other associated brain abnormalities.

Q: What are the treatment options & prognoses for diagnosed hydrocephalus?

Treatment	Examples	Notes
MEDICAL	**Acetazolamide & Furosemide**	Reduce CSF secretion. *Ineffective in long term.*
	Isosorbide	Increases CSF absorption. *Ineffective in long term.*
INTERVENTIONAL	**Serial Anterior Fontanelle CSF Taps (infants).**	Useful in patients with 'transient' communicating hydrocephalus e.g. post SAH. Avoids risks of surgery. *Not practical in long term.*
	Serial Lumbar Puncture (adults – up to twice daily).	
SURGICAL	**Ventriculoperitoneal (VP) Shunt**	Most common procedure. Usually extends from right lateral ventricle (in the right parietal region), to the peritoneum. Prone to blockage (50% <2 years), tubing fracture & infection. *Very effective.*
	Ventriculoatrial (VA) Shunt	Usually extends from right lateral ventricle to jugular vein. Used when abdomen not suitable e.g. peritonitis / multiple abdominal surgery. Rare association with glomerulonephritis. *Very effective.*
	Endoscopic 3rd Ventriculostomy (ETV)	Endoscopic fenestration of 3rd ventricle floor 'creating' new CSF flow channels. Most efficacious in adults with obstructive hydrocephalus (70%). *Less effective than shunts.*
	Ventriculopleural shunt	'Last resort' shunt when Abdomen / cardiac shunt not suitable. Pleural effusion common complication. *Very effective.*
	Lumbar-Peritoneal Shunt	Can be used for benign intracranial hypertension & some types of communicating hydrocephalus. *Very effective in select cases.*

CNS Infections

Q: What are the most common CNS infections?

Remember to consider involved micro-organisms as viral, bacterial, fungal & parasitic. The most common & most significant micro-organisms are bacteria. CNS infections may be broadly classified as cranial vs. spinal:

CRANIAL	Common Bacteria	Notes
Brain Abscess	**Often multiple including:** • *Staphylococcus aureus.* • *Streptococcus milleri.* • *Bacteroides spp.* • *Pseudomonas aeruginosa.*	*(see below)*
Subdural Empyema	• *Streptococcus milleri* >60%. • *Haemophilus spp.* • Anaerobes.	Pus rapidly spreads along the subdural space, but does not cross boundaries e.g. falx cerebri & tentorium cerebellum. **Cause:** Iatrogenic e.g. post -operative. Spread of pus from sinusitis, otitis media & mastoiditis. **Features:** Fever, lethargy, reduced consciousness, focal neurological deficit, seizures in 70% of cases. **Investigations:** Diagnosis may be difficult, even with CT. **Treatment:** As for brain abscess *(see below).*
Meningitis	**Neonates:** • Group B / D *Streptococcus.* • *Escherichia coli.* • *Staphylococcus aureus.* **Infant / Young Child:** • *Neisseria meningitidis.* • *Streptococcus pneumoniae.* • *Haemophilus influenzae.* **Teenager / Adult:** • *Neisseria meningitidis.* • *Streptococcus pneumoniae.* **Trauma / Post-Operative:** • *Staphylococcus aureus.* • *Pseudomonas spp.* • *Enterobacter spp.* • *Mycobacterium tuberculosis.*	Inflammation of the meninges of the brain & spinal cord. **Cause:** • Infection. • Iatrogenic e.g. post-operative. • Chemicals e.g. intrathecal drugs. • Tumour e.g. brain tumour / lymphoma. • Inflammatory sarcoidosis. • Traumatic e.g. penetrating head injury, base of skull fracture. **Features:** Meningism, decreased GCS, focal neurological deficit, sepsis (petechial rash in meningococcal sepsis). **Investigations:** Blood tests e.g. FBC, U&E, CRP. Blood Cultures. CT Brain (excludes mass lesion). LP (*microbiology* - gram stain, MC+S / *biochemistry* - protein, glucose, WCC / *virology* & *immunology* as required). **Treatment:** Resuscitation, broad spectrum antibiotics immediately (gram -ve cover essential), analgesia, possibly corticosteroids, definitive management depends on cause.

CRANIAL	Common Bacteria	Notes
Ventriculitis	• Coagulase -ve *Staphylococcus*. • *Escherichia coli.*	Inflammation of the ventricular cavity & ependymal lining. **Cause:** V/P Shunt, intrathecal chemotherapy, post-meningitis (rarely aseptic). **Features:** Markedly decreased GCS, sepsis, enhancing ventricles on imaging **Investigations:** LP (CSF sample establishes diagnosis). **Treatment:** Intrathecal & intravenous antibiotics until CSF clear. Remove shunt / re-site EVD if present.

SPINAL	Common Bacteria	Notes
Primary Discitis	• *Staphylococcus epidermidis* (most common post-op). • *Staphylococcus aureus.* • *Escherichia coli.* • *Proteus spp.* • *Pseudomonas spp.* (common with IVDU).	Infection of nucleus pulposus, then vertebral body. **Cause:** Iatrogenic e.g. post-operative (0.2–4% incidence after lumbar discectomy). Immunocompromise e.g. HIV, IVDU, DM. Obesity, multiple surgeries & sepsis at time of surgery are risk factors. **Features:** Severe localised pain that is worse on spinal movement, radicular symptoms, tenderness, muscle spasm. Investigations: **Investigations:** Blood tests e.g. FBC, U&E, CRP. Blood Cultures. MRI. Spine X-ray usually normal in 1st week. **Treatment:** Brace, bed rest, analgesia, antibiotics 4–8 weeks, surgery (for associated abscess / unstable spine).

Q: What factors predispose to brain abscess development?

Factors	Notes
Contiguous Spread (most common)	From ENT infection into adjacent brain: • Sinusitis (spreads to inferior frontal lobe). • Mastoiditis (spreads to inferior temporal lobe).
Head Injury	Penetrating Head Injury.
Immunocompromise	HIV, Steroids, DM.
Systemic	Bacterial Endocarditis, Congenital Cyanotic Heart Disease.

Q: What are the common clinical features of brain abscesses?

Most patients present with a history of symptoms <2 weeks:

Features	Frequency	Features	Frequency
Headache	70%	**Nausea & Vomiting**	40%
Mental State Changes	65%	**Seizures**	30%
Focal Neurological Deficit	65%	**Nuchal Rigidity**	25%
Fever	50%	**Papilloedema**	25%

Q: What are the treatment options for brain abscesses?

Medical	Surgical	Follow-Up
Empirical Antibiotics (initially)	Image Guided Burr Hole & Abscess Aspiration (repeat if necessary)	Clinical Progression
Anticonvulsants (>6months)	Craniotomy & Surgical Excision	Serial Imaging
Specific Antibiotics (after MC+S)	Ventricular Drainage (for intraventricular extension)	Serial Inflammatory Markers
Intrathecal Antibiotics (for intraventricular extension)		

Brain Tumours

Q: What are the causes of an intracranial mass lesion?

Classification	Examples
Congenital	Arachnoid Cyst, Hamartoma, Dermoid Cyst.
Infective	Abscess, Toxoplasmosis, Subdural Empyema, Hydatid Cyst.
Inflammatory	Multiple Sclerosis, Reaction Around Foreign Body.
Neoplastic	Primary (Fig 10.8) & Secondary Tumours *(see below)*.
Trauma	Extradural Haematoma, Subdural Haematoma, Intracerebral Haematoma.
Vascular	Aneurysm, AVM, Cavernoma.

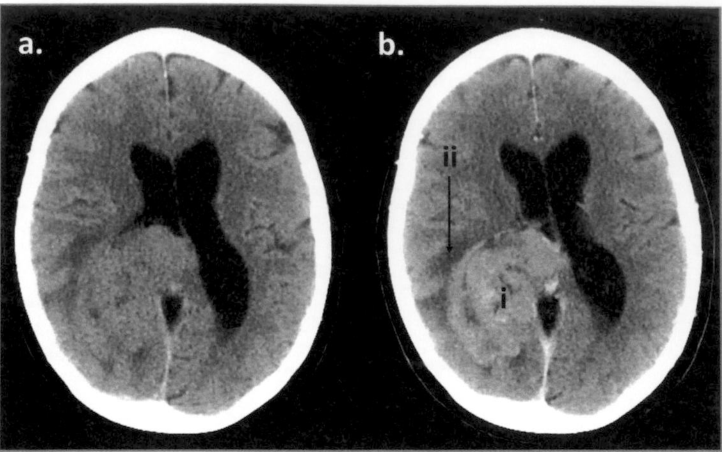

Fig 10.8: Non-contrast (a) & contrast enhanced (b) axial CT brain demonstrating large right parietal enhancing space occupying lesion (i), with extension into the ventricular system. There is surrounding low density that represents oedema (ii). These features are consistent with a malignant primary tumour.

Q: What is the epidemiology of brain tumours?

- Primary brain tumours have an annual incidence of 7.5/100,000 & result in >3,500 deaths/year.
- It is the 15th most common cancer in adults & 2nd most common in children (after leukaemia).
- Metastases account for 50% of brain tumours & prevalence increases with age.
- Metastases are found in 25% of post mortems (with brain examinations).
- Despite modern treatments, primary malignant brain tumours have a poor outcome.
- Outcome for metastatic brain tumours depends on the primary pathology & extent of metastatic spread.

Q: What risk factors are associated with development of a brain tumour?

- Most arise in patients without an obvious predisposing factor.
- <5% are associated with genetic conditions including Von Recklinghausen's Disease (NF1 gene), tuberous sclerosis (TSC1 & TSC2 genes), Li-Fraumeni syndrome (P53 gene).
- Radiation exposure e.g. previous whole brain radiotherapy.
- Immunocompromise e.g. HIV & primary CNS lymphoma.
- Possible increased risk from certain chemical exposures.
- No proven link with mobile phone use or previous head injury.

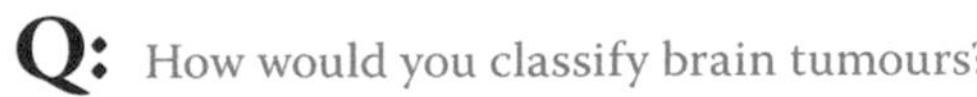

Q: How would you classify brain tumours?

These may be **benign or malignant, primary or secondary** & may be classified **according to location** as follows:

Tumour	Classification		Notes
PRIMARY (45%)	*Intra-Axial (within brain parenchyma)*		
	Glioma (69%)	Astrocytoma (61.5%)	Arise from astrocytes in any part of the brain. Diffusely infiltrative, with ill-defined capsule around tumour. WHO grading 1–4 (increasingly malignant) • Grade 1 (2%): Pilocytic – median age 13 • Grade 2 (23%): Diffuse – median age 40 • Grade 3 (30%): Anaplastic – median age 45 • Grade 4 (45%): Glioblastoma Multiforme – median age 55+
		Oligodendroglioma (5%)	Arise from oligodendroglial cells. 1p19q co-deletion is 'genetic signature'. Frontal lobe involvement common.
		Ependymoma (2.5%)	Arise from ependymal cells e.g. 4th ventricle. 2 peaks of incidence at ages 5 & 35 years.
	Lymphatic (3%)	Lymphoma	Often intraventricular. Increased risk with immunocompromise. May regress with steroids.
	Extra-Axial (outside brain parenchyma)		
	Meningioma (20%)		Arise from arachnoid cap cells. More common in females. Mostly parasagittal (attached to midline) & convex (over hemisphere surface). Slow growing & usually benign.
	Pituitary (5%)		Usually benign adenomas. May present with endocrine hyper- / hypofunction. Bitemporal hemianopia is due to upward compression of the optic chiasm.
	Cerebellopontine (3%)		Acoustic neuroma often presents with sensorineural hearing loss & facial nerve palsy. Usually benign & surgery / radiosurgery is curative.

Tumour	Classification	Notes
SECONDARY	*Intra-Axial / Extra-Axial*	
(50%)	**Metastases**	Small, often multiple, lesions with disproportionately excessive oedema. More common in patients aged >60 years. Most are intra-axial but some are extra-axial (attached to dural surface). Common primary lesions include: • **Lung** (60%): Especially small cell carcinoma. • **Breast** (20%)**:** Oestrogen receptor positivity predicts favourable response to chemotherapy. • **Others** (20%)**:** Colon, melanoma, prostate, renal, testicular.
OTHER	**Vascular**	Haemangioma (Von Hippel-Lindau Syndrome).
(5%)	**Midline**	Dermoid cyst, epidermoid cyst.
	Pineal	Pinealblastoma / pinealcytoma, germ cell tumours.

Q: What are the clinical features of brain tumours?

These depend on the mechanism of involvement e.g. direct infiltration & destruction of neurones, local pressure on neighbouring structures or generalised increase in ICP. Clinical features therefore include:

- Headaches (morning), nausea & vomiting, papilloedema (all due to raised ICP).
- Drowsiness.
- Seizures.
- Focal neurological deficits (depending on location) including:
    - Hemiparesis (contralateral frontal involvement)
    - Dysphasia (Broca / Wernicke involvement)
    - Cranial nerve palsy, cardiorespiratory disturbance (brainstem involvement)
    - Ataxia, incoordination, hydrocephalus (cerebellum involvement)

Q: What are the radiological features of common brain tumours?

These are dependent on the imaging modality & tumour. CT requires pre- & post-contrast scan comparison. MRI demonstrates if metastases are solitary or multiple. Magnetic resonance spectroscopy (MRS) can generate useful information about tumour activity. Common imaging findings are as follow:

Diagnosis	Findings
Glioma (high grade)	Large lesion (often) with central low density (necrosis). Ring enhancement. Rapid progression.
Metastases	Small & multiple (often). Less ring enhancement than glioma. Disproportionately excessive peri-tumour oedema.
Meningioma	Extra-axial. High density on non-contrast CT. Slow progression.

Q: What are the surgical treatment options & prognoses of common brain tumours?

Tumour	Treatment	Prognosis
Glioma	**Grade 1:** Gross total surgical resection ± radiotherapy.	Likely to be curative with total excision, especially in children.
	Grade 2: Surgical debulking depending on location. Chemotherapy has proven benefit.	30% survival at 5 years. 85% transform to a higher grade.
	Grade 3: Surgical debulking depending on location & adjuvant radiotherapy. Chemotherapy has proven benefit.	Median survival 2 years (with treatment).
	Grade 4: Surgical debulking depending on location & adjuvant radiotherapy. Chemotherapy has proven benefit.	Median survival 10 months (with treatment).
Metastases	**Non Small Cell Lung:** Surgical debulking / biopsy & radiotherapy.	Poor prognosis. Depends on resection of primary tumour & other extracranial metastases.
	Breast: Surgery, chemotherapy & radiotherapy.	Can be >5 years with full resection of a solitary brain metastasis & chemosensitive tumour.
Meningioma	Curative surgery is usually feasible even with bone involvement. Radiotherapy indicated for all malignant meningiomas.	>90% cure. 5–10% recurrence if benign. 5% are malignant & have a poor outcome.

CHAPTER 11
UPPER LIMB NERVES

BH Miranda
K Asaad
M Nicolaou
SK Al-Ghazal

CHAPTER CONTENTS

Radial Nerve Examination

Median Nerve Examination

Ulnar Nerve Examination

OSCE Questions

- Radial Nerve
- Median Nerve
- Ulnar Nerve
- Nerve Injuries & Palsies

RADIAL NERVE EXAMINATION

START: Patient sitting opposite you, with hands resting on a table / supported by a pillow.

Expose patient to at least above the elbows. However, some nerve injuries may originate more proximally, so exposing the entire upper limb & cervical spine is ideal.

Look for any aids e.g. splints.

LOOK	Interpretation
Scars	Check for scars indicating penetrating trauma of the upper limb: • Upper arm (fractured humerus) • Radial side of elbow (fractured radial head)
Swelling	Soft tissue / bony mass.
Symmetry	Symmetrical disease is associated with RA.
Deformity	Wrist drop (ask the patient to hold their hands & arms out straight).
Erythema	Inflammation.
Sinus	Post-operative, infective.
Muscle Wasting	Wrist extensors, triceps.

Ask about pain.

Feel for temperature changes (dorsal & ventral) with the back of your hand.

SENSATION	Interpretation
1st Dorsal Web Space	Innervated by the superficial radial nerve.
Dorsal Forearm	High lesion.

Remember to test like-for-like

MOTOR	Interpretation
Triceps	Triceps extension affected with high lesions (nerve branch is proximal to spiral groove).
Brachioradialis	Elbow flexion affected with lesions above the elbow (nerve branch is distal to spiral groove).
Supinator	Supplied by the posterior interosseous branch of the radial nerve (PIN). The PIN branches off at the level of the elbow, passing deep between the 2 heads of supinator.
MCPJ Extension	The radial nerve supplies all long digital extensors.
Extensor Pollicis Longus (EPL)	Patient keeps palmar surface of hand flat on a table & lifts thumb. EPL is usually visible & palpable.

SPECIAL TESTS	Interpretation
Functional Assessment	Assess global & fine function (*see hand examination).*

COMPLETION	Interpretation
Upper Limb Neurovascular Status	Full examinations required *(see relevant sections).* Particularly focus on pulses, dermatomes & myotomes.
Neck Examination	Exclude cervical spine pathology.
QoL Impingement & Sleep	Asking patient about these helps to assess impact on life & therefore necessity for intervention.
Help Patient Dress	Good practice if patient has functional limitation.
Radiology	Humerus fracture (radiograph). Cervical spine (MRI).
Nerve Conduction Studies	Assist in further diagnosis of underlying pathology e.g. degeneration, demyelination, conduction block.

FINISH:

MEDIAN NERVE EXAMINATION

START: Patient sitting opposite you, with hands resting on a table / supported by a pillow.

Expose patient to at least above the elbows. However, some nerve injuries may originate more proximally, so exposing the entire upper limb & cervical spine is ideal.

Look for any aids e.g. splints.

LOOK	Interpretation
Scars	Carpal tunnel decompression / previous trauma.
Swelling	Soft tissue / bony mass.
Symmetry	Symmetrical disease is associated with RA.
Deformity	Benediction sign (when the patient makes a fist), ape hand, simian thumb.
Erythema	Inflammation.
Sinus	Post-operative, infective.
Muscle Wasting	Thenar eminence, forearm flexors.

Ask about pain.

Feel for temperature changes (dorsal & ventral) with the back of your hand.

Feel for reduced sweating.

SENSATION	Interpretation
Thenar Eminence	Innervated by the palmar cutaneous branch, this passes over the flexor retinaculum. It branches from the median nerve proximal to the carpal tunnel.
Digital Nerves	Test all ulnar & radial digital nerves. The median nerve classically supplies sensation to the radial 3½ digits after it has passed through the carpal tunnel.

Remember to test like-for-like.

MOTOR	Interpretation
Pronator Teres	Pronation is affected with high lesions.
Opponens Pollicis	Ask the patient to touch each finger, in succession, with their ipsilateral thumb.
Abductor Pollicis Brevis (APB)	Ask the patient to place their hand on the table (palm up) & point their thumb to the ceiling. Tell the patient to stop you from pushing their thumb down & simultaneously palpate the bulk of APB.
Flexor Pollicis Longus (FPL)	**Pincer Grip:** The patient makes an 'OK' sign with each hand, by pinching their thumb & index finger together. A piece of paper is slipped between the pinched grips of both hands (thumbs facing up). Using your own pincer grips, gently pull the paper away from the patient, asking them to prevent you from doing this. If FPL is affected, the patient's thumb will flatten to prevent the paper from being pulled away. This occurs as the patient switches to using adductor pollicis (ulnar nerve). FPL is supplied by the anterior interosseous nerve (Fig 11.1).

SPECIAL TESTS	Interpretation
Tinel's Test	Carpal tunnel syndrome *(see hand examination).*
Phalen's Test	Carpal tunnel syndrome *(see hand examination).*
Functional Assessment	Assess global & fine function *(see hand examination).*

COMPLETION	Interpretation
Upper Limb Neurovascular Status	Full examinations required *(see relevant sections).* Particularly focus on pulses, dermatomes & myotomes.
Neck Examination	Exclude cervical spine pathology.
QoL Impingement & Sleep	Asking patient about these helps to assess impact on life & therefore necessity for intervention.
Help Patient Dress	Good practice if the patient has functional limitation.
Radiology	Cervical spine (MRI).
Nerve Conduction Studies	Assist in further diagnosis of underlying pathology e.g. degeneration, demyelination, conduction block.

FINISH:

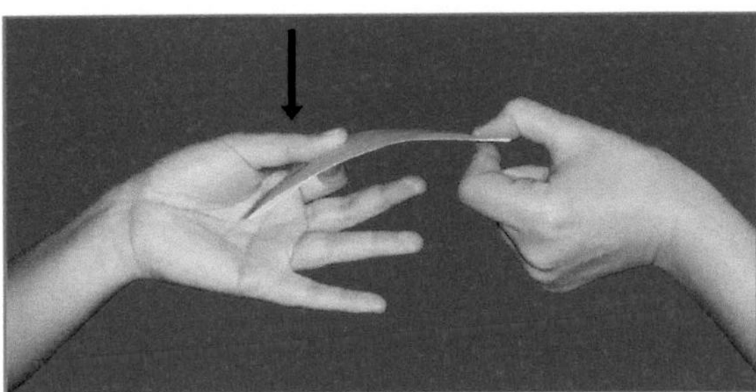

Fig 11.1: Pincer grip test. Flexion at the thumb IPJ is maintained in the normal hand. This is due to the innervation of FPL by the anterior interosseous nerve. On the abnormal hand, adductor pollicis takes over, innervated by the ulnar nerve, such that there is flattening of the thumb (arrowed). Compare with Froment's Test (Fig 11.3).

ULNAR NERVE EXAMINATION

START: Patient sitting opposite you, with hands resting on a hand table.

Expose to at least above the elbows. However, some nerve injuries may originate more proximally, so exposing the entire upper limb & cervical spine is ideal.

Look for any aids e.g. splints.

LOOK	Interpretation
Scars	Cubital tunnel decompression scar posterior to the medial epicondyle / previous trauma.
Swelling	Soft tissue / bony mass.
Symmetry	Symmetrical disease is associated with RA.
Deformity	Claw hand (when the patient extends their fingers).
Erythema	Inflammation.
Sinus	Post-operative, infective.
Muscle Wasting	Hypothenar eminence, Interosseous muscles (intermetacarpal wasting).

Ask about pain.

Feel for temperature changes (dorsal & ventral) with the back of your hand.

Feel for reduced sweating.

Palpate the ulnar nerve behind the medial epicondyle.

SENSATION	Interpretation
All Digital Nerves	Test all ulnar & radial digital nerves. The superficial cutaneous branch of the ulnar nerve classically supplies sensation to the ulnar 1½ digits, via the digital nerves, after it has passed through Guyon's Canal.
Little Finger Metacarpal (dorsal aspect)	Innervated by the dorsal sensory branch. It branches from the ulnar nerve, approximately 1 hand's breadth proximal to the wrist.

Remember to test like-for-like.

MOTOR	Interpretation
Flexor Digitorum Profundus (ulnar)	Test the ulnar ½ of FDP (ring & little fingers), by testing distal interphalangeal joint (DIPJ) flexion.
Palmar Interossei	Get the patient to adduct their fingers, placing a sheet of paper between adjacent fingers. Place the opposite end of the paper between your adducted fingers, tell the patient to prevent you from pulling the paper away, & pull. Palmar interossei weakness will result in the paper slipping from the patient's fingers. **Memory: 'PAD'** The **p**almar interossei **ad**duct the fingers relative to middle finger:
Dorsal Interossei	Test abduction of the fingers against resistance (Fig 11.2). Memory: 'DAB' The **d**orsal interossei **ab**duct the fingers relative to middle finger.
Froment's Test	Ask the patient to put their fists together, making a 'thumbs up' sign with both hands. Put a piece of paper between their thumbs & closed fists & ask them to hold it in place with their thumbs. Adopting the same position, place the opposite end of the paper between your thumbs & closed fists. Tell the patient to prevent you from pulling the paper away & pull. Weakness of adductor pollicis will result in the patient flexing their thumb to prevent the paper being pulled away. This occurs as the patient switches to using flexor pollicis longus (median nerve).

SPECIAL TESTS	Interpretation
Guyon's Canal Percussion	May reproduce ulnar nerve symptoms, if compression is within Guyon's Canal.
Cubital Tunnel Syndrome	Ask the patient to fully flex their elbows & tuck them closely into the sides of their abdomen. Reproduction of ulnar symptoms suggests cubital tunnel syndrome. Percussion over the cubital tunnel may also reproduce symptoms.

COMPLETION	Interpretation
Upper Limb Neurovascular Status	Full examinations required *(see relevant sections).* Particularly focus on pulses, dermatomes & myotomes.
Neck Examination	Exclude cervical spine pathology.
QoL Impingement & Sleep	Asking patient about these helps to assess impact on life & therefore necessity for intervention.
Help Patient Dress	Good practice if patient has functional limitation.
Radiology	Cervical spine (MRI).
Nerve Conduction Studies	Assist in further diagnosis of underlying pathology e.g. degeneration, demyelination, conduction block.

FINISH:

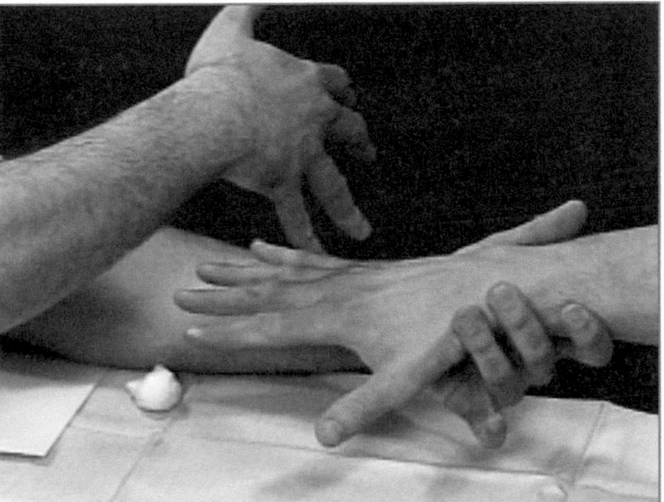

Fig 11.2: Abduction of the little finger, tested like-for-like.

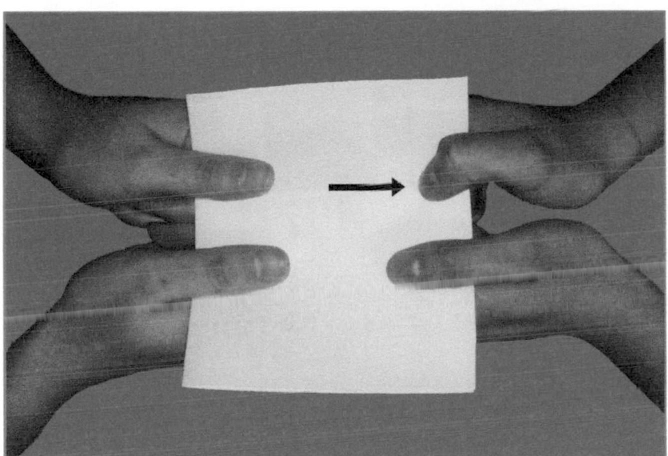

Fig 11.3: A positive Froment's Test. The thumb IPJ flexes to grip the paper. This is due to FPL action (innervated by the anterior interosseous branch of the nerve) taking over from adductor pollicis (innervated by the ulnar nerve). Compare with the pincer grip test (Fig 11.1).

OSCE QUESTIONS

Radial Nerve

Q: What is the course of the radial nerve?

- Roots C5–T1.
- Arises from the posterior cord of the brachial plexus.
- Passes through the triangular space.
- Descends the posterior humerus in the spiral groove between the medial & lateral heads of triceps.
- Gives a nerve branch to **triceps** & **anconeus**.
- Above the elbow it gives a nerve branch to **brachioradialis**.
- At the level of the lateral epicondyle it divides into 2 branches:

Superficial Radial Nerve (superficial branch)	Posterior Interosseous Nerve (PIN) (deep branch)
Descends the dorsal-radial aspect of the forearm, beneath brachioradialis.	Winds around the neck of the radius & passes between the superficial & deep heads of supinator (Arcade of Frohse).
Emerges to a subcutaneous position at the junction of its middle & distal third.	Supplies **wrist extensors & supinators, hand extensors** & **APL**.
Supplies **sensation on the dorsal 1st web space**.	Supplies **ECRL** & **ECRB**.

Q: What is the typical appearance of the hand in radial nerve palsy?

This will depend on the level of injury:

- A high radial nerve palsy results in complete wrist drop due to loss of all extensors.
- A palsy affecting the PIN alone will result in loss of extension of all digits, with preservation of wrist extension (as ECRL is still functioning via the superficial radial nerve). A small patch of sensory loss on the dorsal 1st web space may also be identified.

Median Nerve

Q: What is the course of the median nerve?

- Roots C6–T1.
- Arises from the medial & lateral cords of the brachial plexus.
- Passes with the brachial artery.
- Passes through or under pronator teres & continues beneath FDS.
- Supplies **pronator teres, palmaris longus**, **FCR & FDS.**

- Gives off the **anterior interosseous nerve.** This supplies **FPL**, **radial ½ FDP**, **pronator quadratus.**
- Gives off the **palmar cutaneous branch** 5cm proximal to wrist. This supplies **sensation to the palm of the hand (in line with the radial 3½ digits)**.
- Enters the carpal tunnel & gives off:
    - **Recurrent motor branch** to the **LOAF muscles** (**l**umbricals (radial 2), **o**pponens pollicis, **a**bductor pollicis brevis & **f**lexor pollicis brevis)
    - **Digital cutaneous branches** which supply **sensation to the radial 3½ digits.**

Q: What is the appearance of the hand in a high median nerve palsy?

Appearance	Notes
Thenar Eminence Wasting	Lose innervation to **abductor pollicis brevis, flexor pollicis brevis** & **opponens pollicis.**
Benediction Sign	The index & middle fingers remain extended when the patient tries to make a fist.
Ape Hand Deformity	Wasting of the thenar muscles, results in the thumb coming to lie in line with the remaining digits. Thumb movement is limited to flexion & extension, with loss of abduction & opposition.

Ulnar Nerve

Q: What is the course of the ulnar nerve?

- Roots C8, T1.
- Arises from the medial cord of the brachial plexus.
- Descends the posterior-medial aspect of the humerus.
- Pierces the medial intermuscular septum.
- Passes posterior to the medial epicondyle in the cubital tunnel.
- Passes between the 2 heads of FCU to enter the anterior compartment of the forearm.
- Gives branches to **FCU** & **FDP (ulnar ½).**
- Gives off the **dorsal sensory branch** at the distal ⅓ of the forearm. This perforates deep fascia & runs on the ulnar side of the dorsum of the wrist & hand, supplying **sensation to the dorsal-ulnar aspect of the hand**.
- The ulnar nerve continues through Guyon's Canal (medial to the ulnar artery) & divides into:

Deep Motor Branch	Superficial Sensory Branch
Supplies **all intrinsic hand muscles except LOAF (median nerve).**	Supplies **sensation to the ulnar 1½ digits.**

Q: What is the typical appearance of the hand in ulnar nerve palsy?

- Ulnar clawing of the ring & little fingers.
- This is characterised by MCPJ hyperextension (lumbrical paralysis) & flexion at the PIPJ & DIPJ.
- The clawing becomes more obvious when the patient is asked to straighten their fingers.
- The middle & index fingers are not affected as those 2 lumbricals are supplied by the median nerve (LOAF).

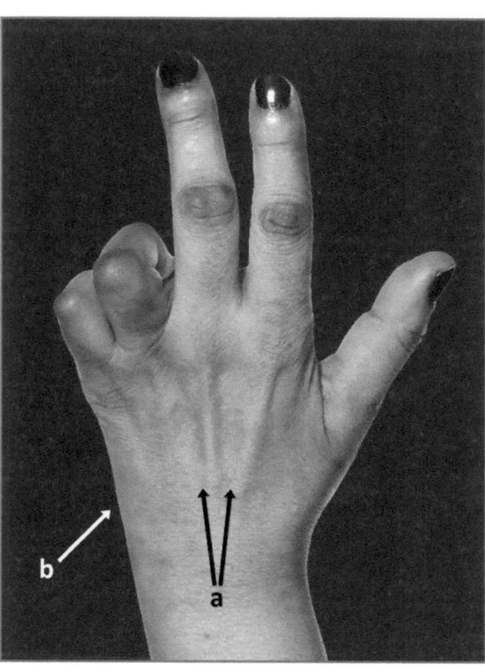

Fig 11.4: A clawed left hand due to ulnar nerve injury. Note the intermetacarpal (a) & hypothenar (b) wasting. There is sparing of the thenar eminence as these muscles are supplied by the median nerve. Compare this with fig 8.2 which shows Dupuytren's Contracture. A thorough systematic examination is necessary to reach the correct diagnosis.

Q: What is the ulnar paradox?

The claw appears worse in a lower (less severe) ulnar nerve injury.

- Clawing is caused because the ulnar 2 lumbricals are paralysed.
  - Lumbricals flex the MCPJ & extend the DIPJ & PIPJ.
- FDP & FDS flex the DIPJ & PIPJ in the fingers.
  - FDP to the ring & little fingers is supplied by the ulnar nerve (flexes DIPJ).
  - FDS is supplied by the median nerve (flexes PIPJ).
- In a high ulnar nerve injury (e.g. at the elbow) there is loss of FDP function, so there is no flexion at the DIPJ & a less-severe looking claw.
- In a low ulnar nerve lesion (e.g. at the wrist) the FDP branch is spared, so flexion occurs at the DIPJ & the claw appears worse.

Q: What is a tardy ulnar nerve palsy?

- Valgus deformity in the area of the medial epicondyle.
  - E.g. caused by malunion / non-union of a condylar fracture.
  - E.g. caused by epiphyseal injury to the lateral side of the elbow.
- Chronic stretching of the ulnar nerve occurs.
- This leads to a late (tardy) ulnar nerve palsy.

Nerve Injuries & Palsies

Q: What are the common sites of radial, median & ulnar nerve compression in the upper limb?

Radial Nerve	Median Nerve	Ulnar Nerve
Thoracic Outlet	Medial Intermuscular Septum	Medial Intermuscular Septum
Axilla	Ligament of Struthers	Cubital Tunnel
Radial Tunnel Syndrome	Pronator Teres	Guyon's Canal
Arcade of Frohse	Anterior Interosseous Syndrome	
ECRB	Carpal Tunnel	
Supinator		

Q: What fractures may be associated with radial, median & ulnar nerve injuries?

- Humeral shaft fractures are associated with radial nerve injuries.
- Median nerve injuries may be associated with wrist fractures.
- Ulnar nerve injuries are associated with supracondylar humeral fractures.
- Phalangeal or metacarpal fractures may be associated with digital nerve injuries.

Q: Can you summarise the effects of nerve injuries in the upper limb?

Nerve Injury		Muscles Affected	Sensory Loss	Appearance
RADIAL	**Axilla**	• Triceps • Brachioradialis • Supinator • ECRL & ECRB • Extensors	1st Dorsal Webspace	• Reduced / Absent Elbow Flexion • Reduced / Absent Supination • Wrist Drop • Absent Digital Extension
	Spiral Groove	• Brachioradialis • Supinator • ECRL & ECRB • Extensors	1st Dorsal Webspace	• Reduced / Absent Supination • Wrist Drop • Absent Digital Extension
	Proximal Forearm	• Extensors	1st Dorsal Webspace	• Milder Wrist Drop • Absent Digital Extension
MEDIAN	**Elbow**	• FDS • FDP (to index & middle fingers) • FPL • FCR • Pronator Teres • Palmaris Longus • LOAF Muscles	Radial 3 ½ Digits & Palm	• Benediction Sign • Ape Thumb
	Wrist	• LOAF Muscles	Radial 3½ Digits	• Ape Thumb
ULNAR	**Elbow**	• FDP (to ring & little fingers) • FCU • Interossei • Ulnar 2 Lumbricals • Adductor Pollicis • Hypothenar Muscles	Ulnar 1½ Digits	• Less Severe Clawing (of little & ring fingers) • Interosseous Wasting • Hypothenar Wasting
	Wrist	• Interossei • Ulnar 2 Lumbricals • Adductor Pollicis • Hypothenar Muscles	Ulnar 1½ Digits	• More Severe Clawing (of little & ring fingers) • Interosseous Wasting • Hypothenar Wasting

SECTION B: COMMUNICATION SKILLS & ETHICS

CHAPTER 12
COMMUNICATION SKILLS & ETHICS

M Epstein
LK McMurray
BH Miranda

CHAPTER CONTENTS

Introduction

Point Scoring

Key Competencies

- Interpersonal Skills
- Information Gathering
- Information Giving & Referral Letters

Ethical & Legal Principles

- Capacity
- Gillick Competence
- Consent
- Advanced Directives
- Organ Donation
- Confidentiality

Communication Skills OSCE Scenarios

- SCENARIO 1: 'The angry patient'
- SCENARIO 2: "Breaking Bad News"
- SCENARIO 3: "Don't tell dad about the diagnosis"
- SCENARIO 4: "Refusal of treatment"
- SCENARIO 5: "Explaining a diagnosis"
- SCENARIO 6: "Organ Donation"
- SCENARIO 7: "Apologise for a mistake"
- SCENARIO 8: "Resuscitation decision"
- SCENARIO 9: "Self discharge"
- SCENARIO 10: "Consent to a trial"

INTRODUCTION

The MRCS OSCE includes dedicated ethics & communication skills stations. However these domains are assessed throughout the OSCE stations, so it is important for an appropriate ethical & communicative framework to be used throughout the examination process.

The stations which specifically test ethics & communication skills can be presented in a variety of formats. The candidate may be expected to role play a scenario with an actor whist being observed by the examiner. Other stations are unmanned e.g. writing a patient transfer letter or filling out an investigation request form. Some example themes & stations include:

Theme	Example Stations
Information Gathering	• Taking a history from a patient. • A consultation with a relative of a patient.
Information Giving	• Writing a patient transfer letter. • Conducting a telephone conversation. • Taking a patient history and presenting it to a consultant. • Completing investigation request forms.
Appropriate & Factual Communication	• Obtaining informed consent. • Breaking bad news. • Discussing investigations. • Discussing a diagnosis. • Discussing treatment options, including complications & relevant prognoses. • Discussing a management plan with a colleague.

POINT SCORING

In order to maximise points, consider the following patient & surgeon factors. These are based on General Medical Council & Intercollegiate Surgical Curriculum Project guidelines.

Patient Factors	Surgeon Factors
Consider age, culture, ethnicity, religion & disability.	Address patients or relatives from a variety of cultural, religious & ethnic backgrounds.
Establish rapport through empathy & honest communication.	Treat all patients, relatives & colleagues with courtesy & respect.
Allow time to listen to the patient's account.	Address a spectrum of pre-existing emotional states of patients or relatives.

Patient Factors	Surgeon Factors
Identify & respond to the patient's or relative's verbal & non-verbal cues.	Address a spectrum of emotional responses from patients or relatives.
Be non-judgemental, non-paternalistic & non-patronising towards the patient or relatives.	Address complaints & questions appropriately, including those beyond the candidate's level of competence.
Respect patients' views about their health, responding to their ideas, concerns & expectations.	Ensure patients are well informed about their care & how their information will be shared within involved medical & surgical teams.
Use a holistic approach to patients & relatives.	Address time constraints.

KEY COMPETENCIES

There are numerous potential scenarios that assess communication skills. The candidate should be prepared to interact with a patient, relative, carer or allied healthcare professional. Although it is impractical to approach the station with a rigid framework, a few competencies will have to be demonstrated:

Competency	Explanation
Interpersonal Skills	• The ability to form a good rapport.
Information Gathering	• Effectively eliciting important information, including ideas, concerns & expectations. • Summarising the patient's agenda to confirm understanding.
Information Giving	• Explaining the issues fully, to a level that is clearly understood. • Avoiding the use of jargon. • Providing an appropriate management plan within the framework of the patient's ideas, concerns & expectations. • Ensuring that summaries are clear & concise if writing a patient referral letter.
Ethical & Legal Principles *(see later)*	• Ensuring the consultation respects the basic ethical principles. • Ensuring the consultation is within the correct legal framework.

Interpersonal Skills

Interpersonal skills are required to build up the doctor–subject relationship. These encompass a number of verbal & non-verbal attributes throughout the consultation:

Interpersonal Skill	Examples
Body Language	• Open body language, avoiding crossed legs or arms. • Maintaining an appropriate distance. • Appropriate, non-threatening eye contact.
Active Listening (verbal & non-verbal)	• Using verbal phrases such as *"Okay..." "Yes..." "I see..."*. • Head nodding. • Echoing the patient.
Empathy	• Using phrases such as *"That must be difficult for you..."* & *"I can see why that must be a problem..."*. • Using silence during the consultation. • Offering a tissue if the subject cries.
Cues Identification & Response	• Responding to verbal & non-verbal cues, which inform you of the patient's needs, desires & feelings. • Using phrases such as *"You mentioned that things were difficult at home, can you tell me more about this?"*.

Information Gathering

The first part of the consultation should be used to elicit the salient points from the subject:

Consultation Step	Explanation	Examples
Introduce	• Use a well-practised phrase. • Give your name to the patient. • Explain your role.	• *"Hello, my name is Dr ... "* • *"I am the surgical doctor on the ward..."*
Check Patient Identity	• Check the name of the patient. • If speaking to a 3rd party, establish their relationship to the patient & ascertain whether the patient is aware of the consultation.	• *"Is it Mr/Mrs ... ?"* • *"Can I ask what your relationship is with Mrs X?"* • *"Does Mrs X know that we are speaking today?"*

Consultation Step	Explanation	Examples
Elicit Reason for Consultation	• Use a well-rehearsed open question. • Do not interrupt the patient as they give their answer. • Listen carefully for cues which you will have to address.	• *"What can I do for you today?"* • *"What is the problem which has bought you here today?"* • *"I'm told you would like to speak to me about Mrs X?"*
Encourage Patient to Provide Information	• Use open questions & active listening techniques to encourage the patient to reveal more information.	• *"Can you tell me a bit more about that..."*

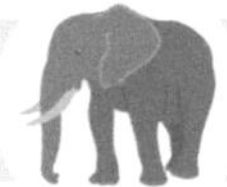

Memory: 'ICE'

It is important to elicit the patient's ideas, concerns & expectations (ICE). This will ensure the consultation is tailored towards the patient's agenda. Marks will be scored if these are identified early in the consultation, reflected upon & applied appropriately.

Consultation Step	Explanation	Examples
Ideas	• What the patient thinks is happening.	• *"What do you know about what has been going on so far?"* • *"What do you think is going on?"*
Concerns	• What worries the patient has that need to be addressed.	• *"Is there anything particular that you are concerned about"* • *"What concerns you most about the current situation?"*
Expectations	• What the patient wants from the consultation.	• *"What do you feel we can do for you today?"* • *"What would you like to achieve from today's consultation?"* • *"How would you like to take this forward?"* • *"What is your understanding of what we are going to do next?"*

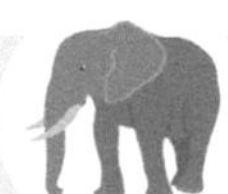

Memory: Summarise!

Before you formulate the management plan, briefly summarise the key points. Summarising demonstrates to the patient that you have listened & understood what they have said. It also demonstrates to the examiner that you have elicited the salient issues & addressed the patient's agenda. You may want to ask:

- *"Can I just summarise what you have told me so far?"*
- *"From what I understand you have told me..."*

After summarising, give the patient the opportunity to divulge any information not picked up during the information gathering process. You may want to ask:

- *"Is there anything else you want to tell me about?"*

Information Giving & Referral Letters

Many communication skills scenarios test the candidate's ability to effectively communicate an explanation & management plan to the patient:

Consultation Step	Explanation	Examples
Explain Issue	• Use simple language. • Avoid medical jargon. • Avoid abbreviations.	• *"Blocked blood vessels"* rather than *"arteriosclerosis"* • *"Do not resuscitate"* rather than *"DNR"*
Ensure Understanding	• Deliver the information in small chunks. • Regularly check that the patient understands your explanation.	• *"Does this all make sense to you so far?"* • *"Do you have any questions about this so far?"*
Formulate Management Plan	• The management plan must be shared. • Avoid being prescriptive, ensure you provide management options to the patient. • Formulate the plan within the patient's ICE.	• *"The options available to us are..."* • *"Are you happy for us to proceed this way?"* • *"We should be able to address your concerns with this test."*
Follow Up	• Arrange a follow up appointment. • Alternatively arrange a contact point for the patient.	• *"I would like to see you in 2 weeks once you have had more time to think about it."* • *"I am on call next week, my bleep number is ..."*
Finish Consultation	• Ask the patient whether they have any further questions. • Always thank the patient.	• "Do you have any questions before we finish?"

Candidates may also be expected to read a set of medical or surgical patient notes & then write a referral or transfer letter to a colleague. Due to time constraints, it is important to gather relevant information from the notes as quickly as possible. Remember that some details may be written down prior to reading through the notes e.g. referring doctor or surgeon details, date, patient details etc. The following information should be included in any transfer letter:

Information	Explanation
Referring Doctor or Surgeon Details	• Name of referring doctor or surgeon. • Details of referring department & hospital. • Contact details.
Referral Date	• Date letter.
Address Referral	• Direct referral with title where possible *"Mr X, Consultant Cardiothoracic Surgeon..."* • An alternative is a speciality referral *"Dear Consultant Cardiothoracic Surgeon..."*
Patient Details	• 1st name, surname, date of birth, age, sex & NHS number
Patient Contact Details	• House number, street name, city & postcode • Include telephone number if possible.
Referral Reason	• Introduce the problem that precipitated the referral. • Ask for an opinion.
Surgical History of Presenting Complaint	• Include onset, duration, course, severity, precipitating factors, relieving factors, associated features & previous episodes.
Other Relevant Medical Details	• Additional current & past medical & surgical problems. • Medications. • Investigation results e.g. blood tests & imaging.
Interpreter	• Mention if required or not.

Here is an example layout for a referral letter:

Mr J Tomkins (A&E SpR)
County Hospital
1 County Street
London L1 1NE
020 7xxx xxxx ext. 1000

Mr H Ali (Consultant Orthopaedic Surgeon)
District Hospital
1 District Street
London L1 1NE
London L1 1NE
020 7xxx xxxx ext. 3000

Referral Date: 21st Jan 2010

Dear Mr Ali,

Re: Jenny Smith, DoB 19/12/1990, Female, Hospital #123456.

Thank you for your kind referral acceptance of the above patient whom I discussed with your ST4, Mr C Jenkins. Ms Smith presented to A&E on the 21st Jan 2010, after sustaining a comminuted fracture of the shaft of the left humerus with shortening & rotation. She sustained this after a mechanical fall onto the edge of a stone step whilst gardening. This was witnessed by her friend who was helping her. There were no other injuries sustained, neither was there loss of consciousness. The patient has no other medical or surgical history & does not take any medication. The AP & lateral view radiographs that were taken are included with the patient notes. No blood test results are currently available for this patient. Ms Smith will not require an interpreter.

Yours sincerely,

Mr J Tomkins

ETHICAL & LEGAL PRINCIPLES

The scenario may be written to test the candidate's ability to identify & appropriately manage an ethical or legal issue.

The four basic ethical principles are:

Ethical principle	Explanation	Example
Autonomy	• Respecting the patient's attitude & wishes with regard to their own health & future.	• Advanced directives. • Do not resuscitate decisions. • Informed consent.
Justice	• Being fair to the wider community in terms of the consequence of a decision.	• Driving after a surgical procedure.
Beneficence	• Ensuring all decisions are **in the patient's best interest.**	• Not undertaking an unnecessary investigation. • Weighing up the benefits & side effects of a medication.
Nonmaleficence	• Ensuring actions **do not harm** the patient.	• Resuscitation resulting in a vegetative state. • Dealing with an unfit colleague.

Capacity

The Mental Capacity Act (2005) provides a framework to assess whether a patient is able to make a decision about their management. This became law in 2007 & applies to anyone over the age of 16. In order to decide if a patient is competent, a number of principles must be followed:

Principles of Capacity	Explanation
Assume the patient is competent unless proven otherwise.	• Do not make assumptions based on appearance, behaviour or current medical condition.
The patient should be in an optimal position to process information & make a decision, prior to assessing capacity.	• Ensure they have adequate time to process the information. • Use appropriate communication aids e.g. interpreters & diagrams.
If competent, the patient has the right to make a decision, even though the decision may be deemed 'unwise'.	• A competent patient may refuse treatment even if it is life saving.
Decisions made on behalf of a non-competent patient must always be **in the patient's best interest**.	• No adult can make a decision for another adult, unless they have lasting power of attorney *(see later)*. • This is regardless of 3rd-party wishes such as family & friends. • Management decisions for non-competent patients must be made by medical or surgical teams & be **in the patient's best interest.**

Assessment of capacity is both decision & time specific. It is only valid for the action being proposed & only for the moment it was taken. A patient's capacity can change over the course of time & from one situation to another.

To prove capacity, the patient needs to demonstrate:

Assessing Capacity	Explanation
Understanding	The patient must understand their: • Condition. • Prognosis. • Proposed management options, including purpose of intervention, risks, benefits & alternatives.
Information Retention	• The patient must be able to retain the information for long enough to make a decision.
Information Evaluation	• The patient must be able to weigh up the risks & benefits of their actions.
Decision Communication	• Communication may include talking, signing or use of any other communication aid.

If a patient lacks capacity, the Mental Capacity Act states:

- Any decisions made must be in **the patient's best interest**.
- The decision should be the least restrictive on the patient's human rights.
- Family & friends can represent the patient's wishes, feelings, beliefs & values, but cannot make a decision on behalf of the patient unless they have lasting power of attorney (see below).
- If the patient has no family or friends to represent them, an independent mental capacity advocate can be appointed.

If a patient lacks capacity, there are 2 situations where a decision can be made on behalf of the patient:

- **Lasting Power of Attorney:** Empowers the patient to appoint an attorney to make health decision for them, if they lack capacity in the future.
- **Court Appointed Deputies:** A deputy is appointed to make decisions, as authorised by the Court of Protection.

Gillick Competence

Patients under the age of 16 are considered to lack capacity unless proven otherwise. When capacity is lacking, parents have the right to make medical decisions on behalf of their child. A patient under the age of 16 who demonstrates capacity, is said to be Gillick competent. There are a number of principles relating to Gillick Competence:

Principles of Gillick Competence	Explanation
Sufficient Intelligence & Understanding	• The child must have a sufficient level of intelligence & understanding in order to process information relating to their management & formulate an informed decision about their treatment. • There must be understanding of the nature, purpose & possible consequences of proposed investigations & treatments. • There must be understanding of the consequences of not having treatment.
Situation Dependent	• Different treatments have varying levels of complexity & life impact, hence they require different levels of intelligence & maturity in order to understand them fully. • If a child is competent to consent for a treatment, their competence should be specifically reassessed prior to a decision about another treatment.
Case-by-Case Decisions	• Each case must be evaluated on its own merit.
Gillick Competent Children's Decisions Can't be Overridden	• Gillick competent children have the right to make an uncoerced decision about their management.

Note: It is important not to confuse Gillick Competence & Fraser guidelines. The latter relates specifically to decisions regarding contraception in minors.

Consent

The candidate should be prepared to fill out a consent form accurately, as part of an unmanned station, or to obtain consent from a patient in a consultation scenario.

Under usual circumstances, consent for a procedure is obtained from a **competent patient with the capacity to make a decision** (discussed earlier). In order for consent to be valid, it must be obtained **without coercion, from a patient who has been well informed** about the treatment options available, including complications & relevant prognoses.

There are 4 consent forms, available from the Department of Health, that apply to various circumstances:

Consent Form	Application
1	Patients able to consent for themselves.
2	Those with parental responsibility, consenting on behalf of a child or young person.
3	Patients able to consent for themselves & those with parental responsibility consenting on behalf of a child, where the procedure does not involve consciousness impairment.
4	Adults unable to consent for themselves.

There are various points in the consent forms that need to be considered by the candidate:

Consent Form Point	Explanation
Patient Details	• These include 1st name, surname, date of birth, age, sex & NHS number. • There is also a space to enter the name of the responsible healthcare professional.
Name of Procedure	• This must be filled in as specifically as possible, avoiding the use of abbreviations.
Benefits of Procedure	• These must be specified. • Examples include diagnosis, symptom improvement & removal of cancer.
Procedure Complications	• These must be specified according to each procedure. • Include the most common & most severe complications only.
Anaesthetic	• GA or Regional Anaesthetic. • LA. • Sedation.
Requirement for Additional Procedures	• Each possible additional procedure must be specified & consented for. • This includes blood transfusion.
Interpreter	• If there is an interpreter present, they must also sign the form.
Patient / Responsible Adult's Signature	• The patient must sign & date the form. • With children, the adult with parental responsibility must sign, though there is a space for the child to sign too, if they so wish. • When adults are unable to give consent for themselves there are spaces for 2 doctors to sign for a procedure that is **in the patient's best interests**.
Capacity	• When adults are unable to give consent for themselves, a capacity assessment must be made that indicates this. • The patient must either be unable to comprehend & retain information, unable to evaluate this information in the decision making process or be unconscious.
Best Interests	• When adults are unable to give consent for themselves, a statement must be made that indicates why the procedure is in the patient's best interests e.g. to save life.
Family Involvement	• When adults are unable to give consent for themselves, it is good practice to involve the family in the management process. They may sign the consent form indicating their approval for treatment. Despite this, they may not override the medical or surgical team's management, unless they have lasting power of attorney.
Medical Signature	• The surgeon undertaking the operation should consent the patient prior to surgery. • In the case of invasive or diagnostic procedures, the doctor undertaking the procedure should consent the patient prior to it.

Advanced Directives

Advanced directives allow competent patients to decide on withdrawal of life-saving treatments should they lose capacity. It can apply to anyone over the age of 18.

The basic principles underlying advanced directives include:

- The patient must have capacity at the time it is created.
- They must not be made under duress.
- They must be signed, dated & witnessed.
- They must specify the circumstances to which they apply.
- Patients can specify treatments to be refused, but cannot demand treatment which are deemed inappropriate.
- Once signed, they cannot be modified verbally or in writing.
- Assuming capacity is present, they can be revoked at any time.

Organ Donation

Absolute contraindications to organ donation include HIV & CJD. Organs can be obtained from either living or deceased donors:

Living Donors
Altruistic donors require mental capacity to be assessed to ensure they are competent to make a decision.
Full informed consent must be obtained prior to donation including success rate, risks to donor & recipient & the requirement for virology assessment.
The Human Tissue Authority must approve all donations from living donors to ensure the decisions were free of coercion or reward.
Living donors can donate their kidney, segment of liver or small bowel.

Deceased Donors
This includes both brainstem death & non-heart-beating donors.
Efforts should be made to ascertain whether the potential donor had expressed a wish to donate.
Evidence includes a written will, donor card, being on the NHS organ donor register or wishes communicated to relatives.
Even if there is evidence of an expression of interest, in practice if the relatives strongly object their views are normally respected.
Relatives of deceased donors are not able to express a preference for the recipient.
Organs which can be donated from deceased donors include heart, lungs, kidney, liver, pancreas, bowel, bone, skin, cornea, face (skin & muscle).

Confidentiality

GMC guidelines state *"Patients have a right to expect that you will not disclose any personal information which you learn during the course of your professional duties, unless they give permission. Without assurances about confidentiality patients may be reluctant to give doctors the information they need in order to provide good care."*

The basic principles of confidentiality include:

- Confidential information should be protected against improper disclosure when stored, transmitted or disposed.
- When a patient has given consent to disclose information, they must be aware of what will be disclosed & the likely consequences.
- Patients must be informed whenever information about them is likely to be disclosed.
- Requests by patients not to submit information to 3rd parties must be respected, unless withholding the information may result in risk to others.
- If confidential information is discussed, only as much information as is necessary to address the issue should be disclosed.
- Health workers should be made aware that the information has been given in confidence.

When confidentiality cannot be breached:

- Casual breaches in & out of the work environment.
- To prevent minor crime or help conviction in minor crime.
- To prevent minor harm to another individual.
- Disclosing information to a 3rd party e.g. insurance company without the patients' consent.

Some situations where confidentiality can be breached:

- Notifiable diseases.
- Drug addiction.
- Births & deaths.
- Court orders.
- When patients who are not medically fit to drive, continue to do so.
- When there is a 3rd party at significant risk of harm. For example, the partner of an individual who has expressed a desire to kill them.

COMMUNICATION SKILLS OSCE SCENARIOS

It is important to practise communication skills scenarios before the OSCE. This allows the candidate to become familiar with the process & timings of the station. The following section provides some example communication skills scenarios. Each case has separate briefings for the doctor & actor. The actor could be anything from a patient to an angry relative.

Practise with a colleague, taking turns between playing the role of doctor & actor. Playing the actor provides valuable insight into how the actor will perceive & respond to the candidate in the exam. If the resources are available, it is useful to have an impartial observer to make notes & give feedback after the consultation.

SCENARIO 1: *"The angry patient"*

DOCTOR BRIEFING

You are the surgical CT2 on the ward & have been managing Mr Bukley, a 65-year-old admitted last night with a critically ischaemic leg. On admission he was found to have:

- Right ABPI - 0.3
- Left ABPI - 0.5
- Absent pedal pulses bilaterally
- No evidence of gangrene or ulcers
- The rest of the cardiovascular assessment was normal
- BP - 138/80
- Blood sugar - 7.8

He was due for an angiogram this afternoon but the procedure has been postponed due to an emergency. It has been rescheduled as the 1st case on the list tomorrow morning. Your consultant has asked you to tell the patient.

ACTOR BRIEFING

You are John Bukley, a 65-year-old retired baker.

Appearance & Behaviour: Anxious, concerned about your condition & upset about the news of the postponement.

Background:

- For the past few years you have had intermittent pains in both legs.
- You saw your GP a few months ago who thought it may be arthritis or a muscle sprain.
- Initially the pain only started after walking about 100 yards but it has been progressively worsening.
- Over the past few weeks you have been getting pain on mobilising a few yards.
- In addition you have been experiencing pain during the night which is helped when hanging the leg out of the bed.
- The pain feels like cramp in the back of your thigh & calf.
- You called an ambulance yesterday evening after the pain became severe & your right foot looked pale & felt cold.
- You were admitted into hospital as an emergency last night.
- After a few tests in A&E you were referred to the surgical doctors who were concerned your leg may not be getting enough blood.
- You were informed of a special test which was urgently required to assess circulation.
- They explained the risks of not getting enough blood to the leg including gangrene & amputation.
- You are currently on the ward.
- You are still in some pain but occasional morphine is helping.

ACTOR BRIEFING

ICE:

- When told of the delay you get angry & are particularly concerned as the doctors in A&E had seemed very concerned about the leg. Why would have they admitted you if the procedure wasn't an emergency?
- You are still in pain & your foot is pale, you feel it may go gangrenous at any time.
- You cannot contemplate living as an amputee; you have seen pictures of amputees from various wars on television.
- Your wife & children are on route to be with you for the procedure, but now you have to tell them that the procedure has been postponed.

Past Medical History:

- You have high BP & are a diet-controlled diabetic.
- You are well otherwise.

Drug History:

- You take a BP tablet called ramipril.
- You have no drug allergies.

Social History:

- You live with your wife in a house.
- You drive & are dependent on your car.
- You started smoking at the age of 22. You stopped about 10 years ago but restarted 5 years ago after retirement.
- You have 2 children who both live nearby.

Family History:

- There is no family history of medical illness as far as you are aware.

First words to the doctor: *"Are you here to prepare me for the procedure?"*

APPROACH TO STATION

Key Principles:

- The station tests the candidate's ability to deal with an angry / upset patient.
- The candidate should aim to diffuse the situation & reassure the patient.
- It is important to be truthful, direct & to apologise sincerely for the current situation.

Introduce Yourself	• *"Hello, my name is Dr ... I am the surgical CT2."*
Check Patient Identity	• Confirm the patient's name. • Check the patient's wristband.
Break News	• Inform the patient that the investigation has been delayed until tomorrow. • Explain the reason for the delay.
Apologise	• The patient may be too angry to acknowledge an apology so be sure to repeat it later in the consultation.
Diffuse Situation	• Let the patient talk & don't interrupt them. • Remain polite & avoid confrontation.
Empathise	• Empathise that you understand why he is anxious about getting treatment as soon as possible.
Identify ICE	• Listen carefully to pick up cues & elicit fears & concerns from the patient.
Address Ideas & Concerns	• Address his fear regarding the immediacy of the investigation. • Reassure him that he is still considered to be high priority by the vascular team. • Ensure he is aware that he is the first case on the list tomorrow morning. • Advise that you are happy to speak to him again with his family when they arrive. • Ensure his pain is controlled as he may need more analgesia overnight. • Suggest that he can speak to the consultant if he wishes.
Summarise & Check Patient Questions	• Summarise the plan. • Offer to answer any further questions.
Close Consultation	• Ask the patient whether they have any questions. • Explain that he can contact the ward doctor at any time. • Thank the patient for their understanding.

SCENARIO 2: "Breaking bad news"

DOCTOR BRIEFING

You are the surgical ST4 in out-patient clinic. Your next patient is Mrs Susan Arnold, a 70-year-old referred with a 2 month history of dysphagia & weight loss. She has undergone a barium swallow which shows an irregular narrowing, highly suspicious of malignancy.

Explain the suspicion to her & the need for a staging CT.

ACTOR BRIEFING

You are Susan Arnold, a 70-year-old retired GP receptionist.

Appearance & Behaviour: You are highly anxious about coming for the results of your test.

Background:

- For the past 2 months, you have been experiencing a sensation of food getting stuck when swallowing & upper abdominal pain.
- You have lost weight (about 1 stone in 6 weeks).
- You went to the GP who was very efficient & sorted out a quick consultation with the hospital doctor.
- You have undergone a test called a barium swallow where you swallowed dye to look at your 'food pipe'.
- You have come for the results of the test.
- Your husband is ill with seasonal flu so unfortunately couldn't attend.

ICE:

- You are worried about cancer but your GP said there were a few possible reasons to explain your symptoms.
- You were a receptionist in a GP surgery & remember a few patients with oesophageal cancer who passed away quickly after diagnosis.
- You wish your husband was with you in the consultation but he is at home with the seasonal flu.
- Your main physical problem at the moment is not being able to eat proper meals because food keeps getting stuck.
- When you are told it looks like cancer, you want to know whether you should call your son back from Australia.

Past Medical History:

- You had your appendix removed at the age of 22.
- You have suffered from irritable bowel syndrome for many years.

ACTOR BRIEFING

Drug History:

- You take occasional mebeverine for your irritable bowel syndrome.
- You have no drug allergies.

Social History:

- You live with your husband who is your "rock" of support.
- You smoked many years ago.
- You drink the occasional glass of wine (about twice a week).
- You have 3 children, 1 in Australia, the other 2 live locally.

Family History:

- There is no family history of medical illness as far as you are aware.

First words to the doctor: *"I've come for the results of my test."*

APPROACH TO STATION

Key Principles:

- This is a breaking bad news station.
- The patient may cry, regardless of your approach.
- Interpersonal skills are particularly important in this station.
- Ensure the patient doesn't sense you are pressured for time.
- Ensure there is adequate support available for the patient.

Introduce Yourself	• *"Hello, my name is Mr ... I am the surgical ST4."*
Check Patient Identity	• Confirm the patient's name.
Initiate Consultation	• Establish whether the patient would like someone to be in the consultation with them.
Elicit ICE	• Establish what the patient knows already about their condition & the test performed. • This will help gauge whether the patient has any insight into the diagnosis.
Break News	• It is always difficult to break bad news. • Ensure you are honest, sincere & give the patient adequate time during the process. • Break the news in small chunks. • Fire a warning shot before mentioning cancer, for example *"I'm afraid the results are worrying"*. • Avoid jargon, mention cancer rather than "growth", "neoplasm" or "malignancy". • Despite the need for confirmatory tests, avoid giving false hope to the patient about an alternate diagnosis. • Advise that there is a strong possibility of cancer but further tests need to be carried out.

APPROACH TO STATION	
Empathic Response	• If there is silence, avoid the temptation to fill it, give the patient a few moments to respond & ensure the consultation pace isn't rushed. • If the patient cries offer them a tissue & allow them to express their emotions. • Be empathetic *"I can see & understand that you are distressed by the news."* • Ask if cancer had been considered by the patient, this will help establish whether the patient had mentally prepared for the news.
Patient Questions or Concerns	• Ask the patient if they have any questions or concerns. • This will help steer the consultation to address the patient' agenda. • The patient may volunteer that she was a medical receptionist & knew a few patients who died of oesophageal cancer.
Explain Plan	• It is important to give a clear plan but avoid giving too much technical information. • Advise the patient of the need for a CT scan & biopsy. • Despite the news, it is important to give hope to the patient about management options. • Mention that there are treatment options including radiotherapy, surgery & symptom-relieving palliation e.g. stents.
Ask About Support	• Ask about family & friends. • Advise of other support networks including the nurse specialist & GP.
Summarise & Check Further Patient Questions	• If the patient is too overwhelmed to think of questions, suggest she can write a list of questions & speak to one of the team or their GP later. • If the patient asks how long they have to live, never give a precise answer. • Ask why they would like to know, there may be a specific reason e.g. wanting to know whether she should call her daughter back from Australia urgently.
Arrange Follow Up	• Arrange a follow up appointment as appropriate. • Leave contact details e.g. bleep number as appropriate.
Close Consultation	• It is important to finish the consultation with a definite plan. • Ensure the patient is safe to travel home. • Thank the patient.

SCENARIO 3: *"Don't tell dad about the diagnosis"*

DOCTOR BRIEFING

You are the surgical doctor, looking after Mr Levent Ali, an 80-year-old man admitted with bowel obstruction. He currently has a naso-gastric tube in situ & is undergoing fluid rehydration. His clinical condition is stable. An abdominal CT scan has revealed a suspicious bowel mass & the appearance of metastatic lesions in the liver. The patient has not been told the news.

The son of Mr Ali would like to have a discussion with you.

ACTOR BRIEFING

You are Mr Imran Ali, the son of Mr Levent Ali. You are 44 years old.

Appearance & Behaviour: You are concerned about your father & feel you know what is in his best interests.

Background:

- Your father has been unwell recently, he has been losing weight & had vomited a number of times before admission to the hospital.
- Since admission the vomiting has stopped & he feels better.
- Currently he is not allowed any food & has had a tube placed into his stomach.
- Your father told you that there may be a blockage in the bowel & a CT scan had been arranged.
- He had the CT scan today but you haven't heard the results yet.

ICE:

- You are suspicious that he may have cancer.
- He has been low in mood for a number of years since your mother died 5 years ago.
- You are concerned that if he finds out about the cancer, he would not cope with the news & sink further into depression.
- He has been in a residential home for the past year & gets carers twice daily who help with meals & bathing.
- He is occasionally forgetful, but you are not concerned about his memory.
- You speak to him every 2–3 days & visit him every weekend.
- Ideally you would like him to go back to the residential home & you will liaise with the GP about managing his further care in the residential home.
- You want to speak to the doctor & get the results of the CT scan before she speaks to your father.
- If it is cancer, you would like the doctor to withhold this information from your father.
- Your father has never mentioned whether he would or wouldn't like to know about a potential serious diagnosis, neither has he mentioned an advanced directive.

First words to the doctor: *"Can I have a quick chat with you about dad?"*

APPROACH TO STATION	
Key Principles: • This station tests the candidate's ability to communicate & negotiate with a relative that has an agenda that differs from yours. • It is important to discuss the issues within an appropriate ethical framework. • The discussion must be balanced & care should be taken to avoid having to deal with an angry relative!	
Introduce Yourself	• *"Hello, my name is Dr ... I am the surgical doctor."*
Check Relationship to Patient	• *"I have been asked to come & talk to you, how are you related to the patient?"*
Initiate the consultation	• Ask an open question such as *"I believe you wanted to have a chat about your father?"* • Actively listen to the son & avoid interrupting him.
Elicit ICE	• Establish what he already knows about his father's condition. • His main concern will be regarding the potential diagnosis of cancer & withholding this information from his father. • Don't be judgemental & try to establish why he has these concerns.
Explain the Difficulty of the Situation	• Be empathic & acknowledge his concerns. • Explain that the CT has been performed, but because of patient confidentiality you should speak to his father first. • Establish whether his father has ever expressed a wish for potentially serious news to be withheld from him. • Explain that if his father were to ask the result of the CT scan, it would not be ethical to lie to him.
Address Concerns & Negotiate	• Try to address the son's concerns & explain why it is important for the father to know the results of the scan. • You cannot consent for any treatment if the patient doesn't know their diagnosis. • If he deteriorates & is unsure of a diagnosis, this may cause him psychological distress. • He may have issues to sort out before he deteriorates further e.g. a will or advanced directive. • Advise that he could ask his father whether he wants to know all the details of his illness & if he chooses not to, you will respect his wishes. • You are happy if the son wants to ask this question of his father. • Reassure him that in your experience, patients like to know their diagnosis & with the right support, cope well with bad news.
Summarise & Check Patient Questions	• Summarise the plan. • Confirm the son understands the issues. • Offer to answer any questions.
Arrange Follow Up	• Arrange a follow up appointment as appropriate. • Leave contact details e.g. bleep number as appropriate.
Close Consultation	• Thank the son.

SCENARIO 4: *"Refusal of treatment"*

DOCTOR BRIEFING

You are seeing Mr Trevor Rogers in urology out-patient clinic.

Mr Rogers is a 54-year-old gentleman with TCC (with carcinoma in situ). He has undergone a course of chemotherapy & radiotherapy but a recent biopsy has shown persistence. He has undergone a CT & bone scan which has shown organ-confined disease.

A recent MDT meeting has concluded that whilst BCG treatment is an option, the approach that would be in the patient's best interests, would be cystectomy with neobladder formation.

The patient is aware of the recent histology results but not the CT & bone scan. Discuss the results of the scan & management plan.

ACTOR BRIEFING

You are Mr Trevor Rogers, a 54-year-old postman.

Appearance & behaviour: Anxious about your diagnosis, but firm about which treatment plan you want.

Background:

- You were diagnosed with bladder cancer 8 months ago after developing blood in your urine.
- You have undergone a course of chemotherapy & radiotherapy but unfortunately the bladder cancer has persisted.
- You had a CT & bone scan & understand that this was to see whether the cancer has spread elsewhere.
- You don't know the results but have come today to get them.
- Your only urinary symptom at present is frequency. You have been told that this is likely due to the chemotherapy & radiotherapy, rather than infection & this may be chronic.

ICE:

- You are concerned the cancer has spread elsewhere & are pleased to hear the results of the scans.
- You are aware that a previously discussed treatment option was removal of the bladder & formation of an artificial bladder.
- You do not want a surgical procedure & are keen to explore all other options before undergoing an operation.
- You have heard of a *"BCG treatment"* & want to know more about it.
- You have a strong belief that even if there is just a small chance of success, you want to try this before losing your bladder.
- You are aware there is a risk the cancer may spread if you choose the BCG treatment, but are firm that this is your preferred choice.
- Currently the cancer doesn't trouble you too much. You work as a postman & occasionally have to find a toilet due to urinary frequency. You are able to carry out all duties.

Past Medical History:

- You are a well-controlled asthmatic, requiring occasional use of the *"blue inhaler"*.

Drug History:

- You are only taking a *"blue inhaler"*, which you don't use often.
- You have no allergies.

Social History:

- You work full time as a postman.
- You have a wife & 2 sons aged 16 & 13 years.
- You do not smoke.
- You do not drink any alcohol.

Family History:

- There is no family history of medical illness as far as you are aware.

First words to the doctor: *"I've come for the results of my test."*

APPROACH TO STATION

Key Principles:

- This station tests the candidate's ability to effectively communicate treatment options within an appropriate ethical framework.
- The candidate should demonstrate to the examiner that capacity is being gauged during the consultation.
- Avoid being judgemental & respect the patient's right to autonomy.

Introduce Yourself	• *"Hello, my name is Dr ... I am the urology doctor."*
Check Patient Identity	• Confirm the patient's name.
Establish Baseline Knowledge	• Ask what treatments he has already undergone. • Confirm he understands why the CT & bone scans were performed.
Explain Scan Results	• Explain the good news that the scans did not show metastases.
Explain MDT Decision	• Explain the MDT's view that cystectomy with neobladder formation is in his best interest. • This decision is based on the previous ineffective chemotherapy & radiotherapy. • Briefly explain the surgical procedure to the patient, avoiding jargon & emphasising that patients cope very well with neobladders.
Elicit ICE	• Listen to the patient's concerns about surgery & preferences for BCG treatment. • Empathise that making the decision about surgery must be difficult for him.
Explain Risks	• Advise that surgery would be curative, whilst a conservative approach would not eliminate the risk of metastasis. • Ensure he fully understands this.
Respect Autonomy	• Mr Rogers is not keen on surgery & is competent to make a decision. • Advise he does not have to make a decision today & can discuss the options with his family or the nurse practitioner. • If his decision is final, ensure you fully support it & avoid being judgemental.
Explain BCG Treatment	• Establish what he knows about BCG treatment. • Explain that the treatment involves catheterisation & introduction of BCG into the bladder through a catheter. • This can stimulate the immune response to attack the tumour. • A number of courses will be required.
Summarise & Check Patient Questions	• Summarise the plan. • Offer to answer any questions.
Arrange Follow Up	• Arrange a follow up appointment as appropriate. • Leave contact details e.g. bleep number as appropriate.
Close Consultation	• Inform Mr Rogers that you will report his decision back to the MDT & they will contact him shortly. • Thank the patient.

SCENARIO 5: *"Explaining a diagnosis"*

DOCTOR BRIEFING

You are seeing Mr Trevor Gregory in vascular out-patient clinic.

Mr Gregory is a 58-year-old gentleman who presented to his GP with abdominal pain. Blood tests were normal apart from a raised ALP of 140. USS revealed a fatty liver & an incidental 4.1cm AAA. The rest of the ultrasound was normal. He has been referred by his GP to the vascular clinic for further assessment of the AAA.

Physical examination is normal.

Explain the findings & the need for surveillance.

ACTOR BRIEFING

You are Mr Gregory, a 58-year-old estate agent.

Appearance & Behaviour: Anxious about the need for referral to the vascular clinic.

Background:

- You went to your GP a few months ago with some intermittent abdominal pains.
- You had some blood tests & were told that a liver test called the "ALP" had come back slightly raised at 140.
- In view of this, your GP sent you for an ultrasound to assess the liver.
- You saw the GP afterwards for the results & were informed that the liver looked a bit "fatty", which might explain the abnormal liver test. However, you were concerned to hear that one of the big blood vessels in your abdomen was enlarged.
- The GP reassured you but advised that you should be assessed by one of the hospital doctors.
- The abdominal pains have resolved & you suspect it may have been due to some stress at work.
- You do not suffer from any back pain.
- You do not have any problems with circulation in your feet.

ICE:

- You have looked up abdominal aortic aneurysms on the internet & are particularly worried that it can burst at any time!

Past Medical History:

- You have high BP. The last reading by the nurse was 160/90. You were told to come back in a few weeks for a recheck but haven't had time due to your job.
- You have high cholesterol & are on tablets.

Drug History:

- You take a drug called ramipril 2.5mg for your BP & simvastatin 20mg for your cholesterol.
- You do occasionally forget to take your tablets.

Social History:

- You work as an estate agent.
- The job has been very stressful recently.
- You live with your wife who doesn't work.
- You have a daughter who is at university.
- You smoke 15 cigarettes a day & have smoked for about 26 years.
- Your wife also smokes.
- You do occasionally think about giving up but due to stress at work, you have not attempted to stop.
- You would consider speaking to the NHS smoking services if suggested.

Family History:

- There is no family history of medical illness as far as you are aware.

First words to the doctor: *"My GP sent me here for assessment of my aneurysm!"*

APPROACH TO STATION

Key Principles:

- The station tests the candidate's ability to communicate a diagnosis & management plan to the patient.
- It is important to assess risk factors & provide appropriate health education to the patient.

Introduce Yourself	• *"Hello, my name is Dr ... I am one of the vascular doctors."*
Check Patient Identity	• Confirm the patient's name.
Establish Baseline Knowledge	• Find out what he knows so far about the USS. • Establish his ideas about the condition.
Explain Investigation Results	• Explain what an AAA is without using any medical jargon. • Give the explanation in small chunks, checking understanding throughout the process. • It may be appropriate to draw a small diagram for the patient.
Elicit ICE	• Establish his concerns, in this case his fear of sudden death. • Make reference to his concerns when explaining the diagnosis & management plan. • Empathise & reassure him that at its current size, the aneurysm only requires monitoring. • Reassure him that there are no other worrying features on examination.
Explain Management Plan	• Advise that he will be closely followed up with 6-monthly USS. • Explain that surgery is considered if the aneurysm increases to over 5.5cm in size, grows >1cm a year or if he becomes symptomatic. • Reassure him that the rupture risk for an aneurysm this size is very low.

APPROACH TO STATION	
Address Risk Factors	• Assess modifiable risk factors including BP, cholesterol & smoking cessation. • Emphasise that addressing these will slow progression of the aneurysm. • Check his compliance with medications & ensure his BP is being monitored. • If he admits to forgetting his tablets, suggest that he builds it into his daily routine e.g. leaving tablets by his toothbrush in morning. • Empathise that it is difficult to quit smoking. Explain that there are services & support groups available. • Explain it is often easier if all smokers in the household give up together. • Advise that he can contact the NHS smoking cessation services.
Summarise & Check Questions	• Summarise the plan. • Confirm he understands the issues. • Offer to answer any questions.
Arrange Follow Up	• Arrange USS in 6 months. • Arrange outpatient appointment.
Close Consultation	• Thank the patient.

SCENARIO 6: *"Organ donation"*

DOCTOR BRIEFING

You have been looking after Mrs Jenny Thomas, a 22-year-old who was admitted with sudden loss of consciousness secondary to a subarachnoid haemorrhage. She has been on a ventilator in the intensive care unit but has recently been pronounced brain dead by 2 attending consultants. You have been asked to speak to her father, Robert Thomas, to inform him of the loss & ask about organ transplantation.

ACTOR BRIEFING

You are Mr Robert Thomas, a 53-year-old accountant.

Appearance & Behaviour: Emotionally upset about the news of your daughter, but prepared for this outcome.

Background:

- You called an ambulance for your daughter yesterday after you found her unconscious in her bedroom.
- Your wife is currently at home but will be coming to the hospital in a few hours.
- The incident was sudden & there was no warning this was going to happen.
- You have been told that she has had a bleed into the brain.
- You are aware that she is not conscious & is on a machine to help her breathing.
- You were told yesterday that the outlook was poor & she may not survive.
- When told she has died you are shocked but had been prepared for the news.
- Jenny has never mentioned her wishes for organ donation in the past.
- She has never carried a donor card.

ICE:

- When the doctor explains the possibility of organ donation, you feel it is a difficult decision to make right now.
- However you do feel Jenny would have wanted to donate organs.
- You would like to know:
    - If you can wait to discuss with your wife?
    - Which organs they may take?
    - You are concerned about face transplant & wouldn't want this to be done.
    - Would organ donation delay the funeral arrangement?

First words to the doctor: *"I believe you wanted to have a chat about my daughter?"*

APPROACH TO STATION	
Key Principles: • The station tests 2 key skills, breaking bad news & discussing organ donation. • It is important to remain empathic throughout the discussion & avoid applying any pressure for a decision on donation.	
Introduce Yourself	• *"Hello, my name is Dr..."*
Check Relationship to Patient	• Confirm this is the father.
Establish Baseline Knowledge	• Find out what the father knows already about his daughter's condition & prognosis.
Break News	• Ask if there is anyone else he would like present. • Explain that unfortunately his daughter has passed away. • Explain that she has been pronounced brain dead & explain what this means. • It is important to emphasise that whilst she is still on a respirator, she has died. • You can explain that if the respirator was to be turned off she would not be able to breathe for herself.
Empathic Response	• Ensure you give time for the father to reflect on the news. • Use silence if appropriate. • Be empathic.
Discuss Organ Donation	• This issue must be approached slowly & tactfully. • Ask the father if he has any knowledge about organ donation. • Explain that organ transplant gives the opportunity to improve the quality of life for other sick people awaiting organ donations. • Empathise that this must be a difficult decision given the current situation. • Explain organs for donation can include heart, lungs, kidneys, pancreas & cornea.
Check if Daughter was in Favour of Organ Donation	• Did they ever have a discussion about organ donation? • Did she carry a donor card? • Did she put herself on the organ donation register? • If donation had never been discussed, what does he think his daughter's views would have been?
Elicit ICE	• Explain he doesn't need to make a decision immediately & has time to talk to his wife about the decision. • Explain that organs are removed in a way to minimise any visible signs on the body. • Advise that the body will be available for the funeral shortly after the organs are removed. • Reassure him that face transplantation has to be specifically agreed upon.

APPROACH TO STATION	
Explain Next Step	• Do not pressurise the father & ensure he knows that his decision will be respected. • If he agrees, explain that you will inform the transplant co-ordinator & the family will be kept up to date throughout the process. • If he decides to wait for his wife, respect this decision.
Summarise & Check Questions	• Confirm he understands the issues. • Offer to answer any questions.
Close Consultation	• Thank the father for his patience & understanding.

SCENARIO 7: *"Apologise for a mistake"*

DOCTOR BRIEFING
You are the ST5 looking after Mr Albert Knox who has had a routine hernia repair. He is recovering but is in pain. He is a type 1 diabetic & normally self administers insulin, however as he is in some discomfort, the nurses are giving his evening dose. Your F1 doctor wrote the insulin dose, but unfortunately due to illegible handwriting on the drug chart, 40 Units of insulin were given to the patient instead of 20 Units. He subsequently had a hypoglycaemic attack which required emergency intravenous dextrose administration by the ward team. Mr Knox has recovered fully & is now alert & well. Mr Knox would like to speak to you about the hypoglycaemic episode. He is unaware of the drug chart error.

ACTOR BRIEFING

You are Mr Albert Knox, a 48-year-old artist.

Appearance & Behaviour: Worried about the recent hypoglycaemic episode & concerned about why it occurred.

Background:

- You have been admitted for a routine hernia repair, which occurred yesterday.
- You are recovering but are in some pain from the operation.
- You are a type 1 diabetic & this evening suffered a hypoglycaemic attack.
- This is strange as your diabetic control is normally very good & you haven't had a hypoglycaemic event for many years.
- At the time you felt sweaty & drowsy.
- You remember a bit of commotion around the ward but had no real insight into what was happening.
- You now feel fine.

ICE:

- You are concerned about why you had the hypoglycaemic event & are keen to discuss this with the doctor.
- When the error on the drug chart is explained, you cannot believe what has happened.
- You are concerned about how the team has cared for you & have lost trust in them.
- You want to know what will happen to the doctor concerned.
- You want to make sure this will not happen again.
- You wish to personally administer your own insulin again.

Past Medical History:

- You are a well-controlled type 1 diabetic, diagnosed at the age of 8 years.
- You have not had a hypoglycaemic attack for many years & are followed up by your GP & the hospital endocrinology department.
- You have not had any previous hospital admissions.

Drug History:

- Apart from insulin you take no other medication.
- You do not have any allergies.

Social History:

- You are an artist.
- You live alone.
- You do not smoke.
- You drink 2–3 glasses of wine a week.

Family History:

- There is no family history of medical illness as far as you are aware.

First words to the doctor: *"I wanted to have a chat with you about my diabetes..."*

APPROACH TO STATION	
Key principles: • The station tests the candidate's ability to be honest with the patient & sincere in apology. • Never lie & do not apportion blame to any particular individual.	
Introduce Yourself	• "Hello, my name is Mr ... I am the ST5 surgeon."
Check Patient Identity	• Confirm the patient's name. • Check the patient's wristband.
Establish Baseline Knowledge	• Ask if he knows what happened to him.
Explain Mistake & Apologise	• Explain that he had a hypoglycaemic attack earlier which required emergency intravenous glucose administration. • Explain that it seems he was given too much insulin by the ward staff. • Advise that this was because an error had been made when interpreting the dosage on the drug chart. • Ensure you apologise sincerely to the patient, accept that there was an error.
Elicit ICE	• Allow the patient to express his concerns & respond to them appropriately. • Advise that medical errors are rare & are taken very seriously. • Do not divert blame onto the nurse or the F1 doctor. • If he expresses concerns about the team, empathise but reinforce that such mistakes are very rare. • Reassure him that the episode will not affect his recovery.
Explain Next Step	• Explain that there is a formal system to ensure the risks of such an error recurring are minimised. • Advise that the consultant will be involved. • Advise that if he is upset he can discuss the issue with the consultant. • If the patient wants to formally complain, explain there is a PALS system which can facilitate this.
Summarise & Check Questions	• Confirm that he understands the complaints procedure. • Offer to answer any questions.
Close Consultation	• Apologise again & thank the patient.

SCENARIO 8: *"Resuscitation decision"*

DOCTOR BRIEFING

You are looking after Mrs Ruby Rose, an 88-year-old lady who has been admitted with a fractured neck of femur (complete fracture with full displacement). She is known to have dementia & has been admitted from a residential home. She is on the operating list for surgery tomorrow. She is currently confused & you have been asked to speak to the son regarding a resuscitation decision.

ACTOR BRIEFING

You are Phillip Rose, the son of Ruby Rose. You are 56 & work in information technology.

Appearance & Behaviour: Concerned about your mother & keen she gets optimal treatment regardless of her age.

Background:

- Your mother has been in a residential home for the past 3 years.
- You were called by the home today & told that she had a fall & was in hospital.
- You have been told that she has a fractured hip.
- At present she is confused & does not seem to understand what is happening.
- She was put into the home a year after your father died because she was suffering from worsening dementia & could not cope alone.
- You had some guilt about putting her in a home, but she has settled & seems content there.
- At the home she can wash & dress herself, but needs supervision.
- She can feed herself & the meals are prepared by the home.
- She walks with a Zimmer frame & has had 2–3 falls over the past 12 months.
- She has been fairly well & active & you feel she has an adequate quality of life.
- She still participates in activities around the home & has friends who she sits with.
- You are unsure on her exact past medical history but you know she has high BP & an irregular heartbeat.
- If asked, you are not sure what tablets she is on but know she is definitely not on warfarin.

ICE:

- When asked about the resuscitation decision you are not happy as you feel she still has a good quality of life.
- You are concerned the team may give her suboptimal care once this decision is made.
- Some of your concerns will be addressed if the doctor explains that the "do not resuscitate" decision does not mean she will receive inferior treatment & that it will only apply if her heart was to stop.
- If she were able to express her wish, you are sure she wouldn't want any prolongation of her life if she were gravely ill.

First words to the doctor: *"How is my mother getting on?"*

APPROACH TO STATION	
Key Principles: • The station requires effective communication of the current situation & prognosis. • Listen carefully to the son's concerns regarding resuscitation & try to address them. • Avoid being prescriptive & try to reach a shared decision.	
Introduce Yourself	• *"Hello, my name is Dr ... I am one of the orthopaedic doctors..."*
Check Relationship to Patient	• Confirm he is the son.
Establish Baseline Knowledge	• Find out what he knows about the current situation & plan.
Empathic Response	• Acknowledge that this is a difficult time for the family.
Explain Plan & Prognosis	• Explain that his mother needs surgery. • Convey the risks associated with surgery.
Elicit ICE	• Ask if his mother had ever conveyed an opinion about resuscitation. • Establish what his current ideas are about resuscitation. • Advise that it is often better to have a clear resuscitation plan to avoid unnecessary distress.
Emphasise that Resuscitation is Unlikely to be Successful	• Mention the poor success rate & outcome. • Advise that resuscitation may cause more harm & distress to her. • Explain it can involve prolonged cardiac massage & even if her heart restarts, she would be unlikely to regain consciousness.
Reassure About the Meaning of "Not For Resuscitation"	• Reassure him that this does not mean his mother will receive suboptimal treatment. • Reassure him that any active medical or surgical problems will be managed regardless of the "do not resuscitate" decision.
Empathic Response	• Be empathic about the situation. • Allow time for a response. • Use silence if appropriate. • Reassure him that he can talk to other family members if he wishes. • Offer the hospital religious or spiritual support services if appropriate. • If he questions the decision, always respect his view & try & establish why he feels this way. • Advise that if his mother's confusion settles, the decision will also be discussed with her.
Summarise & Check Questions	• Summarise the plan. • Confirm he understands the issues. • Offer to answer any questions.
Arrange Follow Up	• Leave contact details e.g. bleep number as appropriate.
Close Consultation	• Thank the son.

SCENARIO 9: *"Self discharge"*

DOCTOR BRIEFING

You are looking after Mr Robert Curren, a 44-year-old gentleman who was admitted yesterday with upper abdominal pain & vomiting. He was diagnosed with acute pancreatitis. This is his first presentation. He drinks half a bottle of vodka a day & this is thought to be the cause.

Blood Tests on Admission:	Amylase – 2000U/l
	LFT & Albumin – Normal
	WCC – 14 x 10^9/l
	U&E - Normal
	CRP – 18mg/l
	MCV – 104fl
Current Observations:	Temperature - 37.8°C
	HR- 98bpm
	BP - 136/72

His is nil by mouth & is having intravenous rehydration. His pain is controlled by pethidine.

He has asked to speak to you on the ward.

ACTOR BRIEFING

You are Mr Robert Curren. You are 44 years old & unemployed. You live alone in a flat.

Appearance & Behaviour: Agitated & keen to leave hospital.

Background:

- You have been feeling generally unwell for the past week & developed severe abdominal pain & vomiting yesterday.
- You called an ambulance & were taken into hospital.
- You had some blood tests & were told you had "acute pancreatitis".
- You had never heard of this condition until it was explained by the doctor. You don't understand how severe acute pancreatitis can be.
- You were told this was likely due to alcohol consumption.
- Since admission, you have been told not to eat & are currently on a fluid drip.
- You were given an injection for the pain & sickness.
- You last received an injection for the pain about 4 hours ago.
- You feel much better now but still have some slight nausea.

ICE:

- You were under the impression that once the pain had settled you could be discharged.
- You don't like hospitals & have decided you don't want to stay in hospital any more.
- You are feeling anxious about not having any alcohol.
- You will be happy to stay in hospital once the risks of self discharge are explained & you are reassured about alcohol withdrawal.

ACTOR BRIEFING

Social History:

- You are unemployed.
- You have smoked 10 cigarettes a day for 20 years.
- You have been drinking alcohol excessively for about 6–7 years.
- You drink about half a bottle of vodka a day.
- You normally start drinking at about midday.
- If you don't drink you do get shakes.
- You know you are drinking too much & have been to the GP to discuss this.
- You realise it is harmful & do have feelings of guilt after a drinking session.
- You were given the number for an alcohol cessation service but did not attend.
- If offered, you will be willing to accept some help.
- You have been depressed since losing your job & the GP has signed you off sick.
- You do not take illicit drugs.
- You have not travelled recently.

Past Medical History:

- You have had occasional episodes of abdominal pain & vomiting in the past but nothing as severe as this.
- You have been to your GP with depression & alcohol dependence.

Drug History:

- You are not on regular medications, but take occasional paracetamol for headaches.
- You have no allergies.

First words to the doctor: *"Doctor, I have to get out of here..."*

APPROACH TO STATION

Key Principles.

This is a difficult station which tests the candidate's ability to:

- Explain a diagnosis.
- Assess competency.
- Explain the risks of self-discharge.
- Address concerns.
- Offer lifestyle advice.

Introduce Yourself	• *"Hello, my name is Dr ... I am one of the surgical doctors."*
Check Patient Identity	• Confirm the patient's name.
Elicit ICE	• The key to this scenario is establishing his concerns about staying in hospital & addressing them efficiently. • Find out what he understands about pancreatitis, including the cause.

APPROACH TO STATION	
Empathic Response	• Convey that you understand how difficult & frustrating it is, being in hospital. • Advise that people are only kept in hospital when absolutely necessary.
Explain Necessity to Remain in Hospital	• Explain his condition has improved because of the fluids & painkillers. • Ensure he understands that unless this continues, the pain & vomiting may recur. • Be clear about the complications & risks of pancreatitis, including death.
Address Concerns About Alcohol	• Empathise that you understand the difficulties in stopping alcohol. • Stress the importance of cessation to prevent pancreatitis & other alcohol related illnesses. • Establish whether he is motivated to stop drinking. • Reassure him that there are some medications which can be prescribed to help with the withdrawal process. • Advise that there are alcoholic support services available.
Explain Self Discharge Procedure	• Advise him that if he does self discharge, he will have to take responsibility for the decision, by signing a legal document.
Assess Competency	• Ensure he has understood all of the information & risks of self discharge. • Ask him to summarise the key points back to you.
On Self Discharge	• Ensure you still "safety net" with advice of what to do if symptoms return. • Encourage the patient to see their GP & advise that a letter will be urgently sent to the GP in advance.
Summarise & Check Questions	• Summarise important points. • Ask the patient if they have any further questions.
Close Consultation	• Thank the patient. • Document in the notes. • Discuss with your consultant.

SCENARIO 10: *"Consent to a trial"*

DOCTOR BRIEFING

You are seeing Mr Gary Stevens in outpatient clinic. He is 61 years old & is being managed for intermittent claudication with lipid lowering therapy, aspirin & exercise. You feel he is suitable for entry into a double-blind randomised controlled trial looking at the effect of a new peripheral vasodilator (treatment X) against placebo. The trial is being carried out in the hospital you are working at. The new drug is to be given for 1 year, with 3-monthly follow up via symptom questionnaires & clinical assessment including ABPIs.

In addition there is a hotline which the patient can call if they have any side effects or questions.

Phase I & II trials have only revealed rare side effects such as rash, ankle swelling & headache. At present the patient is taking simvastatin, aspirin & an ACE inhibitor which he will remain on throughout.

ACTOR BRIEFING

You are Mr Gary Stevens, a 61-year-old working in a paper mill. You live with your wife in a house.

Appearance & Behaviour: Relaxed, interested in your condition & keen for further management.

Background:

- You have come for a routine review of your intermittent claudication.
- You understand that the condition is fairly stable & you have made necessary lifestyle changes including starting medication, weight loss & exercise.
- You do not feel the symptoms are worsening, but still get claudication after about 150 yards when walking uphill.
- It does not significantly affect your activities of daily living but you do find it a nuisance.
- If asked, you do not get leg pain at night.

ICE:

- You are being asked whether you would like to be entered into a clinical trial.
- You have heard of clinical trials in the press & remember a recent case in the papers where participants were severely hurt by side effects from a trial drug.
- You are concerned that you would be used as a guinea pig.
- If explained properly by the doctor, you will be happy to be enrolled, especially because you will be followed up regularly.

Past Medical History:

- You have peripheral vascular disease as described above.
- You have high BP.

Drug History:

- You currently take aspirin, simvastatin & ramipril.
- You have no allergies.

Social History:

- You gave up smoking 2 years ago.
- You do not drink any alcohol.
- You work in a paper mill.
- You live with your wife & are totally independent.

First words to the doctor: *"Hello doctor..."*

APPROACH TO STATION	
Key Principles: • This station tests the candidate's ability to discuss the principles of a clinical trial. • The patient must be fully informed of the risks & benefits of participating. • Ensure the consultation is a discussion & avoid pressurising the patient to participate.	
Introduce Yourself	• "Hello, my name is Dr ... I am one of the vascular doctors."
Check Patient Identity	• Confirm the patient's name.
Explain Agenda	• Tell him you would like to invite him to participate in a research trial. • Explain the aims of the study.
Elicit ICE	• Find out what he knows about clinical trials. • Find out what his concerns are about clinical trials if he indicates that he is worried.
Explain Trial	• He will be given either the trial drug or a placebo for 12 months. • Explain the placebo is to eliminate bias from the study • Which tablet he is given will be selected at random. • Neither he nor the people running the trial will know which tablet he is taking. • He will be followed up regularly to assess his progress. • If he has any problems such as side effects, this will be acted upon immediately. • His identity will be kept confidential during the trial & if the results are published; however registration authorities or the hospital ethics committee may need to see his identity.
Explain Trial Benefits	• He will be monitored more closely than usual. • There is a possibility that his condition will improve, although there is no guarantee. • The trial will be helpful to develop future treatments.
Explain Possible Side Effects	• Explain there may be side effects, as shown in the phase I & II trials. • Reassure him that these have been rare & minor. • Advise that there is a telephone hotline he can call or leave a message on 24 hours a day.
Emphasise Choice	• Explain that participation is voluntary & he can think about the decision. • Advise he can withdraw at anytime during the trial if he wishes. • If he agrees, reiterate that his contribution will be valuable to people with his condition.
Summarise & Check Questions	• Summarise important points. • Ask the patient if they have any further questions.
Close Consultation	• Thank the patient.

SECTION C: HISTORY TAKING

CHAPTER 13
STRUCTURED HISTORY

AD Ebinesan
BH Miranda

CHAPTER CONTENTS

Structured History
Presenting Complaint
History of Presenting Complaint
Past Medical & Surgical History
Drug History
Family History
Social History
Activities of Daily Living
Systems Review

STRUCTURED HISTORY

It is important to have a systematic approach to history taking stations during the OSCE. This ensures that the candidate gathers all of the relevant information, in a slick & efficient manner. It is important to stay focused throughout & avoid diverting from the topic. Here follows a suggested framework & tips:

- Presenting Complaint
- History of Presenting Complaint
- Past Medical & Surgical History
- Drug History
- Family History
- Social History
- Activities of Daily Living
- Systems Review.

PRESENTING COMPLAINT

- Must be in the patient's own words.
- Get the most 'recent' symptoms 1st & number them.*

*If a patient has multiple presenting complaints, or a complicated history extending back many years, it may be better to begin by focusing on the most recent complaint. Continue by numbering other complaints in reverse chronological order & complete the remainder of the history-taking process for each complaint. Numbering in reverse chronological order will assist the candidate in separating which complaints are still part of the current problem, part of a separate problem, or part of the past medical history.

HISTORY OF PRESENTING COMPLAINT

- Start with events leading up to most recent symptoms.
- If the above events are complicated or unrelated, then subcategorise by number & address in reverse chronological order.
- Obtain a concise history, using a protocol such as the one presented below.
- Present your history, in the same order as your protocol.

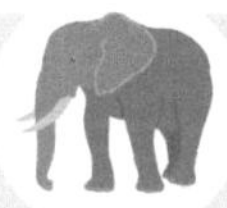

Memory: 'Only Do Clinical Stations, Properly Relaxed & Prepared'

History of Presenting Complaint	Interpretation
Onset	• Did this start suddenly or gradually?
Duration	• When did it start? • How long have you had this for?
Course	• Does it come & go? • Does it get progressively worse? • Is it worse in the morning or at night?
Severity	• How bad is it? • How much would you rate the pain out of 10? *(see box below)* • Does it wake you up at night? • Does it stop you from doing your daily routine? • Does it stop you from working?
Precipitating Factors	• Is there anything that makes it worse?
Relieving Factors	• Is there anything that makes it better?
Associated Features	Ask specifically about the clinical features associated with each system being addressed in the history of the presenting complaint. These are listed in the systems review.
Previous Episodes	• Have you ever had this before?

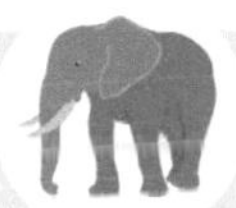

Memory: 'SOCRATES' for pain

If the history of the presenting complaint involves pain, then ask the following:

Site:	Where is the pain?
Onset:	When did the pain start & was this sudden or gradual?
Character:	What is the pain like? An ache? Sharp or stabbing?
Radiation:	Does the pain radiate anywhere?
Associations:	Any other signs or symptoms associated with the pain?
Time Course:	Does the pain follow any pattern?
Exacerbating/Relieving Factors:	Does anything make the pain better / worse?
Severity:	Ask patient to score between 1 (mild) – 10 (severe).

PAST MEDICAL & SURGICAL HISTORY

- Classify this as **medical** or **surgical**.
- It is useful to quickly screen the patient for the following:

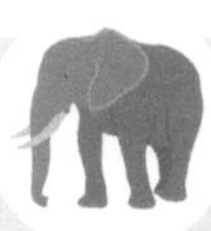

Memory: **'MI THREADS JCAT'**

MI

TB

Hypertension

Rheumatic Fever

Epilepsy

Angina

Diabetes

Stroke

Jaundice

Cholesterol

Atopy (asthma / eczema / hayfever)

Thyroid

DRUG HISTORY

- Don't forget to ask about allergies.

FAMILY HISTORY

- Take a relevant family history only.

SOCIAL HISTORY

- **Accommodation:** Do you live in a house or a flat?
- **Profession:** Are you working? What job do you do?
- **Alcohol:** How many units per week? (limits: ♂ = 21 units & ♀ = 14 units).
- **Smoking:** How many pack years? (20 cigarettes/day for 1 year = 1 pack year).

ACTIVITIES OF DAILY LIVING

- Should be asked in all patients with conditions that may affect function.
- Should be asked in all elderly or frail patients.

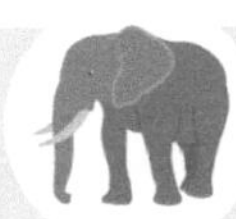

Memory: Remember these according to what your morning routine might be after waking up!

Routine	Activities of Daily Living
Wash	Are you able to wash / bath / shower yourself? Do you need assistance? Do you need hoisting into the bath?
Dress	Are you able to dress yourself? Do you need assistance?
Go Downstairs	Are you able to use stairs? Do you need assistance? How many people assist you?
Cook Breakfast	Are you able to cook? Do you use have deliveries e.g. meals on wheels?
Clean Up	Are you able to clean? Do you need a cleaner?
Use Toilet	Are you able to use toilet facilities independently? Do you need assistance?
Walk Outside	Are you able to walk independently? Do you use a stick or a walker? Do you need assistance? How many people assist you? Do you require use of a wheelchair?
Shopping	Are you able to go to the shops & do your shopping independently? Do you use shopping delivery services? Do you need assistance?
Care Package	Finish by asking if the patient either has a care package already, or requires one. Establish what level of care the patient may already have & assess if the patient is coping with this. If a higher care package is required, communication with a district nurse, the patient's family & relevant support groups is required.

SYSTEMS REVIEW

At the end of the history, the candidate must ensure that a systems review is conducted. This will assist in uncovering any additional problems that may have been overlooked or forgotten during the history taking process.

When addressing associated features during the history of the presenting complaint, the candidate should ensure that all clinical features are enquired about from the relevant system below.

GASTROINTESTINAL	CARDIOVASCULAR
Abdominal Pain	Angina / Chest Pain
Constipation / Diarrhoea	Ankle Swelling
Flatus	Orthopnoea
Haematemesis	Paroxysmal Nocturnal Dyspnoea
Jaundice	Shortness of Breath on Exertion
Nausea / Vomiting	**RESPIRATORY**
Oedema	Chest Pain
Pruritis	Cough & Sputum
Stool Description	Haemoptysis
MUSCULOSKELETAL	Shortness of Breath
Joint Pain / Swelling	**UROLOGICAL**
Loss of Function	Dysuria
Morning Stiffness	Frequency
Power Decrease	Haematuria
Swelling	Incontinence (stress / urge)
Muskuloskeletal Chest Pain	Polyuria / Polydipsia
Associated Urethritis	Poor Stream
NEUROLOGICAL	Terminal Dribbling
Bladder / Bowel Dysfunction	Urgency
Diplopia	Associated Arthritis
Epilepsy / Fits	**GENITAL**
Focal Neurological Defecit	Amenorrhoea
Headaches	Impotence
Hearing Loss	Menorrhagia
Memory Problems	Penile Discharge
Paraesthesia	Period Cycle Abnormalities
Power Decrease	Vaginal Discharge

ABBREVIATIONS

αFP	Alpha Fetoprotein
βhCG	Beta Human Chorionic Gonadotropin
AF	Atrial Fibrillation
AAA	Abdominal Aortic Aneurysm
ABPI	Ankle Brachial Pressure Index
ACE	Angiotensin Converting Enzyme
ACJ	Acromioclavicular Joint
ACL	Anterior Cruciate Ligament
AF	Atrial Fibrillation
AMTS	Abbreviated Mental Test Score
ANDI	Aberrations of Normal Development & Involution
AP Resection	Abdominoperineal Resection
APB	Abductor Pollicis Brevis
APL	Abductor Pollicis Longus
AVF	Arterio-Venous Fistula
AVM	Arteriovenous Malformation
BCG	Bacillus Calmette-Guérin
BP	Blood pressure
Ca	Calcium
CMCJ	Carpometacarpal Joint
CML	Chronic Myeloid Leukaemia
CMV	Cytomegalovirus
CNS	Central Nervous System
CO_2	Carbon Dioxide
CPP	Cerebral Perfusion Pressure
CRP	C-Reactive Protein
CRPS	Complex Regional Pain Syndrome
CRT	Capillary Refill Time
CSF	Cerebrospinal Fluid
CTA	Computerised Tomographic Angiography

CVA	Cerebrovascular Accident
DDH	Developmental Dysplasia of the Hip
DFSP	Dermatofibrosarcoma Protuberans
DIPJ	Distal Interphalangeal Joint
DM	Diabetes Mellitus
DP	Dorsalis Pedis
DVT	Deep Vein Thrombosis
DXT	Radiotherapy
EBV	Epstein Barr Virus
ECRB	Extensor Carpi Radialis Brevis
ECRL	Extensor Carpi Radialis Longus
EDC	Extensor Digitorum Communis
EDH	Extradural Haemorrhage
EHL	Extensor Hallucis Longus
ENT	Ears, Nose & Throat
EPL	Extensor Pollicis Longus
EVLT	Endovenous Laser Therapy
FBC	Full Blood Count
FCR	Flexor Carpi Radialis
FCU	Flexor Carpi Ulnaris
FDP	Flexor Digitorum Profundus
FDS	Flexor Digitorum Superficialis
Fe	Iron
FNE	Flexible Nasendoscopy
FPL	Flexor Pollicis Longus
GCS	Glasgow Coma Scale
GnRH	Gonadotrophin Releasing Hormone
GORD	Gastro-Oesophageal Reflux Disease
HAV	Hepatitis A Virus
HBV	Hepatitis B Virus
hCG	Human Chorionic Gonadotropin
HCV	Hepatitis C Virus
HIV	Human Immunodeficiency Virus
HR	Heart Rate
HSV	Herpes Simplex Virus

IADSA	Intra-Arterial Digital Subtraction Angiography
IBD	Inflammatory Bowel Disease
ICE	Ideas, Concerns & Expectations
ICH	Intracerebral Haematoma
ICP	Intracranial Pressure
IJV	Internal Jugular Vein
IPJ	Interphalangeal Joint
IVC	Inferior Vena Cava
IVD	Intervertebral Disc
IVDU	Intravenous Drug Use
LDH	Lactate Dehydrogenase
LFT	Liver Function Tests
LMN	Lower Motor Neuron
LOAF	Lateral (Radial) 2 Lumbricals
	Opponens Pollicis
	Abductor Pollicis Brevis
	Flexor Pollicis Brevis
LSV	Long Saphenous Vein
MCPJ	Metacarpophalangeal Joint
MDT	Multidisciplinary Team
MRA	Magnetic Resonance Angiography
MRV	Magnetic Resonance Venography
MMS	Mini Metnal State Examination
Na^+	Sodium
NGT	Nasogastric Tube
OA	Osteoarthritis
OT	Occupational Therapy
PCL	Posterior Cruciate Ligament
P_aCo_2	Partial Pressure of Arterial Oxygen
PEG	Percutaneous Endoscopic Gastrostomy
PEJ	Percutaneous Endoscopic Jejunostomy
PFL	Patellofemoral Ligament
PIN	Posterior Interosseous Nerve
PIPJ	Proximal Interphalangeal Joint
PR	Per Rectum

PT	Physiotherapy
QoL	Quality of Life
RA	Rheumatoid Arthritis
ROM	Range of Motion
RR	Respiratory Rate
RTA	Road Traffic Accident
SAH	Subarachnoid Haemorrhage
SCFE	Slipped Capital Femoral Epiphysis
SCJ	Sternoclavicular Joint
SCM	Sternocleidomastoid
SDH	Subdural Haematoma
SFJ	Sapheno-Femoral Junction
SPJ	Sapheno-Popliteal Junction
SSV	Short Saphenous Vein
STD	Sexually Transmitted Disease
SUFE	Slipped Upper Femoral Epiphysis
SVC	Superior Vena Cava
TA	Tibialis Anterior
TB	Tuberculosis
TCC	Transitional Cell Carcinoma
TFT	Thyroid Function Tests
THC	Tetrahydrocannibinol
TIA	Transient Ischaemic Attack
TP	Tibialis Posterior
TPN	Total Parenteral Nutrition
U&E	Urea & Electrolytes
UMN	Upper Motor Neuron
USS	Ultrasound
UTI	Urinary Tract Infection
V/P Shunt	Ventriculoperitoneal Shunt
VL	Vastus Lateralis
VMO	Vastus Medialis Obliquus
VV	Varicose Veins
X-ray	Radiograph
ZN	Ziehl-Neelsen

INDEX

Abdomen 22, 30, 54–6, 83, 95, 114, 146, 178, 200, 214, 248
Abdominal Aortic Aneurysm (AAA) 55, 57, 58, 62, 80, 106, 146, 151–3, 181, 248, 249
Abdominal Regions 58
Abdominal Scars 76
Abducent Nerve 170
Abductor Pollicis Brevis (APB) 138, 174, 212, 217
Achilles Tendon Rupture 120, 121, 133, 134, 178
Actinic Keratosis 8–9
Activities of Daily Living 261, 266, 269
Adhesive Capsulitis 131
Adson's Test 102–3, 154
Advanced Directive 231, 235, 243, 244
Allen's Test 146
Amputation 131, 141, 146, 147, 155, 161, 237
Ankle 20, 58, 105, 114, 116, 118, 119, 120, 121, 147, 151, 174, 175, 178, 180, 183, 261, 270
Ankle Brachial Pressure Index (ABPI) 147, 149, 150, 237, 261
Ankylosing Spondylitis 71, 104, 105, 127–9, 181
Annular Pulley 143
Anterior Interosseous Nerve 174, 212, 213, 215, 217, 219
Ape Hand 211, 217, 220
Apprehension-Relocation Test 109
Apprehension Test 109, 118
Arterial Examination 146–7
Arterial Insufficiency 150
Ascites 57, 63–5
Babinski 178
Bad News, Breaking 224, 240–2, 244, 252
Bamboo Spine 128
Beevor's Sign 105
Bell's Palsy 38
Bell's Reflex 38
Benediction Sign 211, 217, 220
Bouchard's Nodes 123, 136
Boutonniere Deformity 125, 136, 139
Brachioradialis 174, 210, 216, 220
Bragard's Test 105
Brain Abscess 199, 201, 202–3
Brain Tumour 201, 203–7
Branchial Cyst 30, 31, 36
Breast xxiii, xxiv, 7, 22, 46–51, 206, 207
Breast Cyst 50
Budd-Chiari Syndrome 62–3, 65, 67
Buerger's Angle 146
Buerger's Test 146
Bulbocavernosus 179
Campbell de Morgan Spot 8–9
Capacity 231–5, 247
Caput Medusa 54, 64
Carbuncle 10
Carotid Artery Aneurysm 22, 32
Carotid Artery Stenosis 156
Cauda Equina Syndrome 106, 127, 165, 179, 182–5
Cerebellar Signs 173
Cerebrospinal Fluid (CSF) 186, 187, 189, 195, 198–200, 202
Cervical Rib 30, 32, 101, 153
Chemodactoma 30
Chronic Renal Failure 68
Cirrhosis 36, 49, 59, 62–5, 67
Clark's Test 118
Claw Hand 213, 218, 220
Claw Toes 120, 133–4
Clonus 174, 179
Club Foot 120, 133–4
Clubbing 54, 59
Cobblestones 70
Colostomy 94–6
Communication Skills xix, xxii, 223–62
Confidentiality 236, 244, 262
Consent xxiii, 89, 224, 231, 233–6, 244
Contrecoup 190
Contusion 190, 192
Coordination xx, 173, 175, 184, 206
Coup 190
Cranial Nerves Examination 169–72
Cremasteric 86, 178
Crohn's Disease (CD) 55, 69–72, 94
Cruciate Pulley 143
Cryptoglandular Sepsis Theory 74
CT Brain 51, 186, 191, 195, 201, 204
Cubital Tunnel Syndrome 214
Cyclical Nodularity & Mastalgia 49–50
Cystic Hygroma 30, 31
Deep Vein Thrombosis (DVT) 157–9
Deep Venous Insufficiency 158–9
Deltoid 107–9, 120, 174
Dermatofasciectomy 141
Dermatofibroma 8–9
Dermatome 102, 109, 111, 115, 119, 121, 139, 175–7, 180, 183, 211, 212, 214
Dermoid Cyst 30, 203, 206
Discitis 181, 202
Dorsal Column 176
Dorsal Interossei 174, 214
Drug History 238, 241, 246, 249, 254, 259, 261, 266, 268
Duct Ectasia 49–50
Dupuytren's Contracture 54, 136, 137, 218
Dupuytren's Disease 140
Dysdiadochokinesia 173, 175
Dysphagia 21, 26, 28, 60–1, 240
Dysphasia 169, 206
Elbow xxi, 100, 102, 107–11, 113, 136, 139, 173, 174, 178, 180, 210, 211, 213, 214, 216, 218, 219, 220
Epididymal Cyst 82, 89
Epididymitis 82, 88, 90
Epigastric Mass 62
Epistaxis 42
Epithelial Hyperplasia 49, 50
Ethics 224–62
Excessive Breast Development 49
Exomphalos 85
Extensor Pollicis Longus (EPL) 138, 210
Extradural Haematoma (EDH) 188, 190–1, 203
Facial Nerve 23, 36, 37, 38, 171, 205
Facial Nerve Palsy 37, 205
Family History 126, 238, 241, 246, 249, 254, 266, 268
Fasciectomy 141
Fasciotomy 141
Fat Necrosis 51
Felty's Syndrome 67, 125
Femoral Hernia 78, 82, 84
Fibroadenoma 49, 51
Finger–Nose Test 175
Finkelstein's Test 138
Fistula 23, 26, 63, 68, 71, 72–5, 96, 194
Flexion Deformity 104, 110, 113, 114, 117, 120, 133
Flexor Digitorum Profundus (FDP) 138, 143, 214, 217–18, 220
Flexor Pollicis Longus (FPL) 138, 174, 212–15, 217, 220
Flexor Tendon Sheath 143
Foot 20, 105, 118, 119–21, 122, 133–4, 140, 147, 174, 176, 178, 183, 237, 238
Froment's Test 213–5
Frozen Shoulder 131
Furuncle 10
Gait 112, 116, 122, 130, 173, 199
Ganglion 8, 142
Gangrene 94, 136, 146, 161, 237
Garrod's Pads 137, 140, 141
Gastroschisis 85
Gerber's Test 109
Gillick Competence 232–3
Glasgow Coma Scale (GCS) 168–9, 186–7, 190, 192, 201, 202
Glioma 12, 37, 205, 207
Glossopharyngeal Nerve 172
Goitre 5, 18–19, 21, 26, 27–8, 60
Golfer's Elbow 111
Goodsall's Rule 77
Groin Lump 78, 82
Guarding 54, 57
Guyon's Canal 213, 214, 217, 219
Hallux Rigidus 129–30
Hallux Valgus 120, 133–4
Hammer Toes 120, 133–4
Hand 54, 102, 126, 136–44, 146, 154, 211, 213, 216–18
Head Injury 85, 169, 185–9, 192, 199, 201, 202, 204
Head Lymph Nodes 33–5
Heberden's Nodes 123, 136
Heel–Shin Test 175
Hepatic Asterixis 54
Hepatomegaly 62–3
Hernia 6, 8, 31, 54, 58, 62, 78–85, 90, 94, 95, 181, 188, 189, 253, 254
Hip xxiii, 104, 105, 113, 114, 116, 119, 122, 129, 174, 178, 180, 256
History of Presenting Complaint 229, 266, 267, 270
H-Manoeuvre 170–1
Hydrocephalus 198–200, 206
Hydrocoele 82, 87, 90
Hypersplenism 67
Hypoglossal Nerve 25, 172
Ideas, Concerns, Expectations (ICE) 225, 227, 239, 249, 257
Ileostomy 72, 95, 96

Implantation Dermal Cyst 31
Inflammatory Bowel Disease (IBD) ix, 59, 69–74
Information Gathering 224, 225, 226–28
Information Giving 224, 225, 228–30
Infraspinatus 107–9
Inguinal Canal 78, 81–3
Inguinal Hernia 58, 78, 82–4, 90
Interpersonal Skills 225, 226, 241
Intracerebral Haematoma 188, 190, 203
Intracerebral Haemorrhage 190, 192, 193, 195
Intracranial Haemorrhage (ICH) 190–2
Jobe's Test 109, 132
Kayser-Fleicher Rings 55
Keratoacanthoma 8, 10
Kidney 57, 67, 68, 73, 125, 235, 252
Knee 116–19, 124, 147, 178, 180
Koilonychia 54
Lachman's Test 118
Laryngocoele 32
Lasègue's Test 105
Ledderhose's Disease 140
Leg Length 104, 112, 113, 114
Leukonychia 54
Lhermitte's Sign 105
Light Touch 176
Lingual Nerve 25
Lingual Thyroid 26
Lipoma 8, 14, 32, 36, 51, 62, 73
Low Back Pain 127, 181, 182, 184
McMurray's Test 118
Median Nerve 111, 137, 138, 174, 211–219
Meningioma 12, 205, 207
Meningitis 37, 66, 199, 201, 202
Multiple Endocrine Neoplasia 29
Myotome 102, 109, 111, 115, 119, 121, 139, 174, 180, 211, 212, 214
Naevus 8, 11
Neck xv, xix, xxiii, 4, 5, 6, 10, 11, 13, 18–41, 55, 101–3, 105, 109, 113, 171, 199
Neck Dissection 35
Neck Lymph Nodes 33–5
Neer's Test 109, 132
Nerve Compression 130, 153, 219
Nerve Injuries & Palsies 137, 170, 210, 211, 213, 218–20
Nerve Roots 105, 106, 154, 174, 180, 182, 183
Neurofibroma 12, 37
Neurofibromatosis 12
Neuroscience xv, xix, 166–207
Oculomotor Nerve 170
Odynophagia 40, 60, 61
Olfactory Nerve 170
Opponens Pollicis 212, 217, 273
Optic Nerve 12, 170, 205
Orchitis 82, 88, 90
Organ Donation 235, 251–2
Orthopaedics xxiv, 4, 100–134, 154
Osler-Weber-Rendu Syndrome 55
Osteoarthritis (OA) 104, 110, 111, 113, 114, 116, 117, 118, 122, 123–4, 130, 131, 132, 133, 136, 181
Paget's Disease 46, 48, 51, 123, 129–31
Paget's Sign 6
Palmar Interossei 214
Papilloma 13, 51, 199
Parotid Gland 23–4, 31, 36–7
Past Medical & Surgical History 229, 256, 266, 268
Patella Tests 117, 118
Patella Tracking 116
Peau D'Orange 46
Perianal Abscess 74
Periductal Mastitis 49, 50
Perthe's Test 148
Peutz-Jegher's Syndrome 55
Peyronie's Disease 54, 140
Phalen's Test 138, 212
Pharyngeal Pouch 26, 31, 32, 60, 61
Pincer Grip 138, 212, 213, 215
Plummer-Vinson Syndrome 60, 61
Polycystic Kidney Disease (PCKD) 67, 68
Portal Hypertension 63–4, 68
Posterior Drawer Test 118
Posterior Interosseous Nerve (PIN) 174, 210, 216
Posterior Sag Sign 118
Power Grading 174
Presenting Complaint 266–7
Prolapsed Intervertebral Disc 104, 105
Pronator Teres 212, 216, 219, 220
Proprioception 173, 176
Pyogenic Granuloma 13
Radial Nerve 137, 174, 210–11, 212, 213, 216, 219
Radial Nerve Palsy 216
Ramsay Hunt Syndrome 38
Raynaud's Syndrome 154–55
Referral Letter 225, 228–30
Reflexes 20, 106, 170, 173, 178, 179, 180, 184
Retrosternal Goitre 18, 26, 60
Rheumatoid Arthritis (RA) 36, 39, 67, 107, 110, 112, 116, 117, 120, 121, 123, 125–6, 133, 136, 143, 155, 210, 211, 213
Rheumatoid Nodules 111, 125, 136, 137
Rinne's Test 172
Romberg's Test 173
Roo's Test 102, 103, 154
Rose Thorn Ulcers 70
Schober's Test 105
Scrotal Lump 79, 80, 82
Sebaceous Cyst 14
Seborrhoeic Keratosis 8, 11, 12
Sensation 12, 21, 24, 25, 47, 90, 106, 109, 123, 150, 173, 175, 176, 184, 213, 216, 217, 240
Shifting Dullness 57
Shoulder 107–9, 131–2, 174
Sinus 73, 100, 101, 199, 201, 202
Sjögren's Syndrome 36, 39
Social History 238, 241, 266, 268
Spermatocoele 82, 89
Spinal Accessory Nerve 35, 172
Spine xix, 81, 101, 104–6, 107, 112, 114, 115, 116, 128, 173, 182, 186, 202, 210, 211, 212, 213, 214
Spinothalamic Tract 175
Spleen 57, 66–7
Splenomegaly 66–8, 125
Stensen's Duct 23
Sternomastoid Tumour 31
Stoma xiv, 94–6
String Sign 70
Stroke (CVA) 196–8
Structured History 266–70
Student's Elbow 110, 111
Subarachnoid Haemorrhage (SAH) 68, 192–200, 251
Subclavian Artery Aneurysm 22, 30, 32, 154
Subdural Empyema 201, 203
Subdural Haematoma (SDH) 188, 190, 191, 203
Superficial Radial Nerve 210, 216
Supinator 178, 210, 216, 219, 220
Supraspinatus 107–9, 131, 132
Swan-Neck Deformity 125, 136
Systems Review 267, 270
Talipes Equinovarus 133–4
Tardy Ulnar Nerve Palsy 111, 219
Tennis Elbow 111
Teres Minor 108, 109
Testicular Maldescent 82, 86
Testicular Malignancy 90–2
Testicular Torsion 89–90
Testicular Tumour 86, 90, 92
Thomas's Test 113–15
Thoracic Outlet Syndrome 32, 102, 146, 153–4, 219
Thumb Squaring 136
Thyroglossal Duct Cyst 18, 26, 30, 31
Thyroglossal Fistula 26
Thyroid 18–22, 26–34, 59, 101, 130, 268
Thyroid Cancer 27–9
Tinel's Tarsal Tunnel Test 121
Tinel's Test 212
Tone 27, 106, 173, 184, 186
Tonsillitis 40–1, 60, 61
Tourniquet Test 148
Trendelenberg Test 112, 114, 115, 122, 148
Triceps 174, 178, 180, 210, 216, 220
Trigeminal Nerve 130, 170, 171
Trigger Finger 143
Triple Assessment 47, 51
Trochlear Nerve 170
Troisier's Sign 55
Two-Point Discrimination 138, 176
Ulcer 7, 14, 15, 55, 61, 69, 70, 71, 119, 146, 148, 151, 237
Ulcerative Colitis (UC) 69–72
Ulnar Nerve 111, 137, 154, 212, 213–15, 217–19
Ulnar Paradox 218
Umbilical Hernia 85
Undescended Testis 86
Vagus Nerve 172
Varicocoele 82, 89
Varicose Vein 4, 148–9, 159–60
Vascular xix, xxiv, 4, 6, 7, 11, 13, 62, 67, 68, 73, 94, 102, 106, 130, 146–61, 181, 193, 203, 206, 239, 248
Venous Hypertension 158–9
Ventriculitis 202
Vestibulocochlear Nerve 172
Vibration 176
Virchow's Node 55
Von Recklinghausen's Disease 12, 204
Warthin's Tumour 37
Weber's Test 172
Wharton's Duct 25
Xanthelasma 55, 146
Zolen's Test 118
Z-Thumb 125, 136, 139